Touching the Ends
of the Earth

The Story of
Medical Service Ministries

Other titles published by
The Missionary School of Medicine

Decachords (Homoeopathic *Materia Medica*)   Dr. John Clarke
Homoeopathy in Tropical Diseases   Dr. Edwin Neatby
The Bible and Homoeopathy   Ronald R. Male

It is the author's wish that any surplus arising from the
sale of this book be devoted to the publisher's charitable objects.
MSM is a publisher without commercial motive.

The name of the Charity changed on 2 July 1990 to:

Medical Service Ministries
P O Box 133, Ware SG12 7WJ, UK
tel/fax: +44 (0)1920 486039
email: resources.msm@btopenworld.com
Registered Charity No. 234037

Touching the Ends of the Earth

The Story of
Medical Service Ministries

Founded in 1903 as the
Missionary School of Medicine

Philip Price

Editor: Anthea J. Cousins

First published 2003 on behalf of the author
by Medical Service Ministries
P O Box 133, Ware, Hertfordshire, SG12 7WJ, UK

British Library Cataloguing in Publication Data
A catalogue record for this book is available from
the British Library.

ISBN: 0-9509097-3-4

Typeset by Profile, Culmdale, Rewe, Exeter,
produced for MSM by Jeremy Mudditt Publishing Services, Carlisle,
and printed and bound in Great Britain by
Nottingham AlphaGraphics

This book is dedicated to the memory of

Canon A Timothy Houghton M.A.

Former student of the MSM in 1923-1924
Pioneer Missionary in Myanmar (formerly known as Burma)
Longest serving President of the MSM (1948 - 1977)
a Great Missionary Statesman and a Man of God

Contents

Evaluations from Students
from the Ends of the Earth

Queenie Adams	Egypt	72
Margaret Bartlett	Solomon Islands	102
Edward Bingham	Nigeria	44
George Burford	China	28
Mildred Cable	Tibet	50
Ernest Cartwright	Congo	6
Christine Cheal	Nigeria	39
Frank Davies	India	39
Mary Eccles	South India	47
Evelyn Eglington	Peru	100
Kathleen Singleton Fisher	Belgium Congo	11
Elizabeth Flemming	Sierra Leone	131
Sue Frampton	Ghana	131
Raymond Guyatt	Hong Kong	84
Barry Haigh	Zambia	110
Fiona Haines	Djibouti	127
Jenny Hearne	United Kingdom	112
Carla Hein	Indonesia	101
A.Timothy Houghton	Upper Burma	18,39,81
Agnes Hubbard	Morocco	12
Bryn Jones	Brazil	90
Walter Kendrick	Nassau	64
Sharon Liu	China	142
Alfred Lodge	Northern Nigeria	78
Raymond Lower	China and Japan	117
Frances Lyons	Nigeria	90
Sam Mattix	Laos	93
Len Moules	Northern India	29
Dennis Nichol	Angola	58
Philip Price	Kenya	78
Kenneth Richardson	Kenya	58
Emily Rowntree	Angola	108
David Ryan	Brazil	131
Gottfried Schalm	Northern Nigeria	65
Sister Schrader	Solomon Islands	58
Patricia Sills	(not recorded)	82
Charles Tett	Nigeria	1
Mrs Vollrath	Turkestan	19

List of Illustrations

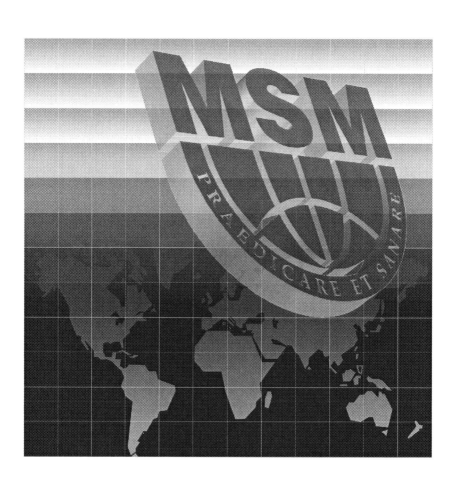

Foreword

The trustees of Medical Service Ministries acknowledge the debt of gratitude owed to Canon Philip Price for the work he has undertaken on their behalf. They believe the writing of this account of the lives of so many, whose gifts and energies have been devoted to the service of our Lord and Saviour Jesus Christ, will bring glory to God. That alone has been their motive in laying this burden upon him.

Philip's involvement, first as a student, then as a missionary, later as a fellow trustee, enabled him to write with understanding and empathy. It is the story of an effective partnership between specialists at the top of their professions and workers aspiring to equip themselves for the Master's service.

In the final chapter and in the appendices I have brought, Philip's account up to 2003, MSM's centenary year.

The trustees look to the Lord for clear guidance and strong faith, believing there is much to be accomplished before He returns.

Brian H.T.Weller

Each of you has been blessed with one of God's many wonderful gifts to be used in the service of others. So use your gift well. If you have the gift of speaking, preach God's message. If you have the gift of helping others, do it with the strength that God supplies. Everything should be done in a way that will bring honour to God because of Jesus Christ, who is glorious and powerful for ever. Amen

(I Peter 4: 10-11) CEV.

Preface

Nothing of importance happened today
Such was the entry in the diary of King Louis XVI of France on 14 July 1789.

Yet on that day in Paris, armed workmen joined forces with civic militiamen and two detachments of French Guards in an all-out bid to seize the Bastille, the hated fortress-prison in the heart of that city. This singular event sparked off the French Revolution which changed completely the future history of that country. The King remained curiously inactive in the face of the crisis, apparently believing that Paris was experiencing another in a series of troublesome bread riots.

Nothing of importance happened...
Looking back over the past century some may be tempted to feel that nothing of importance happened in 1903. How wrong they would be. In that year two remarkable things happened which transformed the overseas mission of the worldwide Church. One was the invention of the aeroplane and its first flight. The other was the founding of what is today known as Medical Service Ministries, but formerly called The Missionary School of Medicine or just the MSM.

Four flights above a north Carolina beach in the USA, on a cold and windy morning in December 1903, each lasting less than a minute, realized a centuries-old dream of flying like birds. This amazing invention spearheaded enormous development, making it now possible for speedy travel in comfort and safety to every part of the globe. Everyone knows of this progress as it has become a normal feature of daily life even in the most remote areas.

On the other hand, so little is known about MSM. And, what *is* recorded stands every chance of being forgotten. This is due to advances in medical practice, and especially to development in Third World countries, which have now largely eliminated the need for the type of training developed by the Missionary School of Medicine.

Preface

However, in its new role and under its new name it continues to offer financial and practical help to mission candidates and workers who seek healthcare and additional medical training for service in many countries.

For those who are and have been involved in its life, it is an amazing story and the Christian world of today is the poorer without a written record of its history. It has been the purpose of this research to try and redress this need.

This is not the first attempt to write the history of the School. Some years ago, the late Miss Lyle Bottom, Warden and Secretary, compiled a most comprehensive history and for comment and advice passed it to a certain individual who failed to return it. Sadly, he could not be traced and she had no copy. So sure was she that this account would eventually be written that MSM received a significant gift from her Executors for this purpose.

The author of this present work was himself a student in the 50th Jubilee Session from 1952-53 before going to serve as a pioneer missionary in Kenya under the auspices of the Bible Churchmen's Missionary Society, now known as Crosslinks. Whilst in that country he was able on many occasions to put into practice some of the several abilities he learnt while a student at the MSM. More recently, he served as a member of the Council of the MSM.

In the early years of its life, the President of the School, Dr. J. Stuart Holden, gave students, as they were commissioned for overseas service for the Master, a little 'Thought' which was repeated each year at the Annual Meeting. It developed into a kind of slogan, *'You are touching the ends of the earth!'* and forms the fitting title for this record, now completed after many years of patient work in the midst of a busy retirement.

The author would like to thank many who have given him assistance in his task. Firstly, the members of the Council of the MSM who asked him to attempt this. He is grateful for their patience over many years of waiting.

Preface

Particular members of that Body deserve a special mention; Mrs Jean Hayward-Lynch for her constant assurance and encouragement, and for lending him the Annual Reports covering much of the last century, from which most of the information in this account was culled; Mr. Brian Weller for his practical help, offering many suggestions and Dr.Anita Davies for reading the first draft of the book with meticulous care and offering much constructive advice, and especially for her contribution in allowing use of her paper in Appendix C.

The Monitor of that Jubilee Session in 1952-53 was Mr. John Brown and the author is greatly obliged to him for writing most of chapter 6, and for the joy of re-discovering his friendship after more than forty years since we parted company in 1953. The author would also like to express his thanks to a recent President, the Rev. T. Omri Jenkins, for his most gracious encouragement at a time when the author was on the verge of giving the whole thing up.

Finally, his greatest thanks are given to his dear wife Grace, for her constant patience over these years and particularly for reading all the manuscripts of the final version and making numerous constructive comments.

Now the author's hope is that many will enjoy reading this account and give much praise to the Great Physician, the Lord and Saviour Jesus Christ, who still commissions His disciples to *'Go into all the world'* and to *'Preach and Heal'*.

Chelmsford
January 2002

1 Beginnings

A Talented Young Missionary

One day in 1943 Charles was left alone in a busy mission hospital in Nigeria. The doctor had been called out to a serious case and both English nurses were ill in bed. Other men might have found something less demanding to do until the situation regained a degree of normality. As a young missionary he could have done some language study, or gone into the bush to do some village preaching; or he could have spent time in the mission school, as he was to do many years later in Kenya, heading up an Industrial Training Centre in the back streets of Nairobi. **Charles Tett**, however, was no ordinary fellow, as we shall discover a little later. He remained in sole charge at that hospital until the doctor returned.

This is how he described the experience:

I had a busy time! I had to take the **morning clinic** with the aid of an interpreter and to do the **ward round**. I felt a little diffident at first but I had read up all I could. Three **emergency** cases came in - one was a threatened abortion, another a septic thigh which was opened and a pint-and-a-half of pus drained off, the third was a stricture. Doctor was quite pleased when he returned and questioned me about my MSM training. He was apt to be rather suspicious because of its **homoeopathic** bias, against which he is quite prejudiced.

I have had much and varied **medical** work since I came to Africa. First I spent a month at the Mission Hospital (**which was allopathic**). Here we were mainly occupied in giving injections for sleeping sickness, dysentery and leprosy. They were very short staffed owing to the war and so **I helped in the theatre where I gave the anaesthetics** for a time. During my stay the hospital was full and overflowing and it gave me an excellent opportunity of **studying tropical diseases** at first hand.

Since arriving at my station, **the medical work** has been handed over to me and I am much encouraged at this form of service and with **the usefulness of homoeopathy**. Already I have one or two cases to report. One was a boy of 8 who came to us bleeding copiously from every orifice and with a badly ulcerated mouth. I hardly knew what to do, but after consulting Boericke (Homoeopathic Materia Medica with Repertory) decided to give him Lachesis. The result was truly remarkable: the bleeding stopped an hour after the first dose and two days later there was only blood in his stools. The ulcerated mouth was improving too, but a dose of Mercurious Corrosivus solved this problem and within a week he was discharged cured.

Another evening, a runner came in from a distance with news of a snake-bite case. The girl's nose was bleeding and they could not stop it. I sent three doses of Lachesis immediately and next day I heard that she was making a good recovery. A week later, I was trekking in the district and saw the girl. On examination of the scar I saw that the wound had cleared up completely and that no sepsis had followed as is usually the case. I might add that three people in this neighbourhood, who were previously bitten, had died through severe haemorrhage.

On **the surgical side**, septic fingers, teeth extractions, hydroceles etc. are very common, so are bad eyes, and ulcers of the leg. Cancrum oris is also very prevalent. I have seen three severe cases recently, besides many others which would have got to that extreme stage, if they had not come to us in time.

Pulsatilla has a great reputation in these parts for prolonged labour and I have had one or two cases to attend to in the midwifery line. I send a big 'Thank you' for all I was able to learn at the MSM. **I don't know what I should have done without it!**

The reader will have noticed several words in bold characters in Charles' gripping letter. This has been done in order to emphasize the varied nature of the training given at the **M**issionary **S**chool of **M**edicine.

The MSM was Born at the Dawn of the 20th Century
After recounting the heroic work and sufferings of the pioneers of the Universities' Mission to Central Africa, the author of the Mission's history wrote:

One ... practical result cannot be overstated. By an experience bitter beyond all possible expectation, the missionary had learnt the lesson that carelessness of life and ignorance of the precautions for preserving health, is not wise for this world or the next; that none, however strong, can afford to play with a tropical climate; that certain rules of health must be kept; and that to remain needlessly in a hotbed of fever, slighting the proper remedies, is not trusting, but tempting Providence. These first missionaries had the bitter lesson to learn. To some extent they could not foresee these dangers and did not know the necessary precautions. But now that the lesson has been deeply scored on that page of Church history, those who neglect its warnings will die...

(History of the UMCA 1897)

Slowly this warning began to be heeded and the enthusiasm and desire to obey the command of our Lord to 'Go and make disciples of all nations...' was tempered by the importance of being adequately equipped for every kind of possible emergency. So it was that in the first two or three years of the 20th century different members of the staff of the London Homoeopathic Hospital began to receive applications from missionaries to be allowed to see some of the treatment being carried out there. They either wrote from abroad, or when on furlough, called to ask for some tuition. In particular were two members of the London Missionary Society stationed in Matabeleland and Mashonaland. They had been brought face to face with illness and accident with which they had been unable to cope. They were shown some of the work in the Out-Patient department and the wards, but the teaching was scanty, scrappy and without system.

The Real Beginning

In the year 1903 the newly formed British Homoeopathic Association undertook to organize systematic instruction for missionaries with regular lectures and practical experience. To Dr George Burford, then Physician for the diseases of women at the LHH (London Homoeopathic Hospital), belongs the credit of suggesting and supervising the foundation of the MSM. Dr Edwin Neatby acted as the Honorary Secretary from its inception.

Comprehensive Instruction

Reporting at the Coming of age celebration 21 years later, Dr Neatby said:

> **The School was not founded with the idea of advancing any particular medical doctrine because its basis was wider than any sectarian or individual basis could be. The School was unique as it sought to press into service every sort and kind of useful curative agent. It did not matter whether this was called by the name of anti-pathy, allo-pathy, or homoeo-pathy, but at this hospital they had the satisfaction that the homoeopathic principle, as one of the great laws of medical practice, was exemplified in the result of their teaching all over the world. They had no cause to regret having kept homoeopathy as one of the important parts of the education.**

Aims of the School

In 1936 Sir John Weir, the Honorary Treasurer, spoke of the aims of the School as being mainly three-fold:

1 To enable missionaries to look after their own health.
2 To enable them to nurse and treat one another on the mission field when ill or miles away from medical aid.
3 To enable them to start dispensaries for the local people and so open the door for the gospel tidings.

It has always been the concern of the best of Christian missionary endeavour to fulfil Christ's command to preach and heal, so as to minister in love to the needs of people everywhere, in body, mind and soul.

The First Session

The first session in 1903 had an enrolment of 24 students. Not all were free to do the whole course but as this facility became known it was soon clear that a real need had been met by the foundation of the School. Applications came from a wide area. The Revd Stuart McNairn was the first registered student. He subsequently served in Peru and later became the General Secretary of EUSA (Evangelical Union of South America), as well as being on the General Council of the MSM. One of his fellow students was Eldred Hercus from New Zealand, a graduate in Arts and a Bachelor of Science; he worked in South America. So also, in the same year, was the Hon. Florence MacNaghten from the CMS Hospital at Peshawer, in Northwest India, where she was the superintendent of nursing. Florence was a keen and capable student, gaining much from the course.

Instruction and practical help was given in all sorts of medical and surgical practices. Students began with anatomy and physiology before going on to hygiene, nursing and bandaging, first aid, and the elements of surgery, medicine, tropical diseases and tropical hygiene. They also received instruction in the treatment of children's diseases and infant welfare work, and last but not least, they became very proficient in extracting teeth.

In far away places, giving a patient relief from bad toothache can bring quick appreciation. Sir John Weir, a Scotsman with a ready wit, loved to tell the story of a man who went to a dentist in Scotland and had a tooth extracted. It took only a few seconds and he asked the dentist, 'How much for that?'

The dentist replied, 'A guinea.'

'But you have only been a few seconds', said the man.

'All right', the dentist replied, 'The next tooth I take out for you, I will hang on for half-an-hour and charge you the same fee!'

It is not known how soon the patient returned!

General Running of the School

The Board of Management of the LHH gave the movement every facility. Both teachers and students had the advantage of using the clinical resources of the hospital. From the start, the project met with the support of almost the entire body of the medical and surgical staff of the hospital by whom most of the instruction was given. At first it was necessary to go to other institutions for the theory and practice of dentistry, and Mr R.J.Lovett and Mr Russell Grant were the first lecturers in this subject. Dr Hawkes travelled from Ramsgate to give lectures in first aid, and Dr Edith Neild came from Tunbridge Wells to provide the lectures in midwifery to the women students.

In those early days, most of the teaching staff would accept only a nominal honoraria, which in many cases would barely cover the fare of a Hansom cab; the prevalent vehicle in those times. In later years also, many of the lecturers declined any such acknowledgment, while others returned their fees. This generosity rendered the work of the Honorary Secretary much easier than it would otherwise have been.

The student's fees were 12 guineas for the full course, and 5 guineas for a single term. Variable amounts were charged for different single subjects.

Appointment of Officers

At first, the arrangements were supervised by the British Homoeopathic Association but it was soon found desirable to appoint independent officials in the shape of President, Vice-President, a General Council and a Medical Executive Committee. It was felt that the work would be helped if influential, missionary-spirited, non-medical men and women could be interested and become involved in this training project.

The Name of the School

Originally, the name chosen was The London Missionary School of Medicine. Later, this was shortened by the omission of 'London' in order to avoid confusion with The London Missionary Society. This shortened title was not only more convenient but quickly gave rise to the acronym - **MSM** - and so it has popularly been known ever since!

Answering Criticisms

From its inception, there were critics against this kind of limited medical training for lay people; such comments as, *'a little knowledge is a dangerous thing'* were sometimes voiced, with the assumption that a little medical knowledge might be worse than no knowledge at all. An argument against a partial medical training was that if at home one would not hand over a sick friend to the care of a person with only limited medical knowledge, why then should one do it abroad? This criticism was answered in such a way as reflected the needs of large parts of the globe, which at the turn of the 20th century was largely unexplored. Some of those answers were as follows:

(a) In China there were districts with a population as large as London without a single doctor with *real* medical knowledge. The local doctor, untrained according to familiar western standards, was still content to puncture a diseased area with rusty needles, or to scarify it to let out an evil spirit, or 'suddenly shut down the lid of a box' to keep it in!

(b) In many parts of Africa it might have taken as long to get the services of a doctor as it would have taken to travel to London from Edinburgh and back ten times! Also, in many parts of this huge continent the people were dependent on the incantations of the witch doctor and were more liable to be killed by a 'Trial by ordeal', or if old and useless, to be thrown out into the forest to die, or be devoured by a lion or leopard.

(c) In India, China or Africa, patients, white or coloured, could die of cholera or other acute diseases in a few hours, before a doctor could reach them.

(d) Prevention is better than cure and a large proportion of the diseases which afflicted missionaries and their converts were preventable.

A student at this time was **Ernest Cartwright**, who later served in the Congo with the Regions Beyond Missionary Union. Speaking some 20 years later at an annual meeting of the School he recalled some of the professional opposition there had been to instructing lay missionaries in medical practice. The whole thing seemed to Ernest to be a matter of *degree*. He would not himself have attempted a serious brain operation, nor would he have tried a laparotomy or some of the more serious operations which were undertaken so lightly by professionals such as Dr Neatby, but that did not seem to him to be any argument why he should not try to do simple things which he had been taught how to do in the LHH when on the course. The important thing was for a person to know how far to go; the things which *could* be done and those which should *never* be attempted, and with that rider it could be safely said that the MSM training was extremely valuable for any missionary, not only to help the sick nationals, but also to look after their own health, and that of colleagues around them.

He went on to say that he had always worked on the assumption that sooner or later he would be alone in a distant land facing medical difficulties that no one but God could help him to meet. He had recently been in that situation. For 17 months he had lived more than four day's journey from the nearest European, making him totally dependent upon the knowledge he had gained from the MSM. For that reason he was particularly appreciative of the practical teaching and facilities allowed him as a student in the classes, at the clinics, and on the wards, in dentistry and in the use of anaesthetics and a full understanding of homoeopathic remedies.

The School Justified

What could students expect to do upon completion of the course in those early years? If a good answer could be given to that question, then in spite of all the opposition from some quarters of the medical profession the existence of the Missionary School of Medicine was more than justified. This is how the School answered that question when it 'came of age' in 1924:

> In surgical work they can dress a wound in a leg, apply a splint for most simple fractures. They know what to do with a clean cut, and from their knowledge of antiseptic and aseptic surgery are likely to get better results with a compound fracture than an experienced surgeon 45 or 50 years ago would have been expected to obtain. They can stop simple bleeding and can tell the difference between arterial and venous haemorrhage.
>
> They know the use of many surgical instruments and know how to profit by books and experience in a way that before their training would have been impossible. If they have had a course of dentistry they can at least extract a tooth without 'the aid of a skewer and a hammer'(!!) and probably can fill a decaying tooth, or at any rate dress it, and so relieve pain until it can be filled.

Medically, they can treat a case of cholera or simple diarrhoea, give correct doses of quinine for fever, prescribe and administer morphia, if necessary, without poisoning the patient, and tackle a case of attempted suicide from opium in China or India. They can make a poultice, or an invalid's bed. They know how to give Aconite after a chill and Antimonium Tartaricum for pneumonia; when to give Belladona for a sore throat and when not to give it.

By this it will be seen that our teaching is on no narrow or sectarian lines. The fact that we teach surgery which is the common ground of all schools of medical thought, that we give systematic instruction in First Aid to the injured, that we have a course of General Therapeutics and yet do not neglect to teach our students as much of homoeopathy as can be learned in one session, constitute sufficient evidence of the catholicity of our training.

Throughout almost the whole of the 20th century many hundreds of students from all over the world enrolled at the School to benefit from the instruction and medical facilities it offered so as to better enable them to go forth into a needy world in the name of their Lord Jesus Christ, to preach and heal. That, more than anything else, is the best testimony to the founding of the Missionary School of Medicine.

2 Early developments

Handbook for Students

In the early days of the MSM one of the very real problems faced by the students was the fact that almost all the medical and surgical text books available were far too technical and advanced for the understanding of those with rather limited experience. For this reason it was decided to compile a handbook mainly for MSM students which would give a clear statement of the causes and transmitting agents of tropical diseases, the symptoms and course, and the prevention and treatment. Difficult technicalities were omitted, or included only where they contributed to a clearer understanding of the subject under consideration. The treatment described included all that was of known usefulness, both general and homoeopathic.

Under the title *A Manual of Tropical Diseases for Missionaries,* its publication was made possible by the generosity of the Honyman Gillespie Trustees and the cordial cooperation of the publishers, Bale Sons and Danielson of London. The book received favourable reviews.

The Museum

Another feature from which the School benefited about this time was a small museum located on the top floor of Hahnemann House in Powis Place leased to the School at a very moderate rental. Dr S.H.Daukes OBE, of the Wellcome Bureau of Scientific Research, regularly conducted students around the bureau's unrivalled Museum of Tropical Diseases, explaining such points as could be of practical use to them. These visits proved so helpful that the Executive Committee of the School decided to try to form a similar, though obviously much smaller museum on its own premises, in order to demonstrate the salient practical features of the hygiene, sanitation and diseases of hot countries.

In the formation of this many groups assisted with help and advice, most notably Dr Newman, the then Director of the London School of Tropical Medicine, Dr Stephens of the Liverpool School of Tropical Medicine, and the Curator of the Museum of the Royal College of Surgeons, Edinburgh and their respective staffs. The first honorary Curator of the MSM Museum was William Watson MD, FRCSI, DTML, who had recently returned from medical missionary service in China and Japan.

Later, when the School celebrated its Coming of Age in 1924, a £1,000 appeal was launched at the Annual Meeting to finance the continued usefulness of this project.

Taking the 'Body' to Pieces!
The task of providing suitable diagrams and models for teaching purposes occupied the attention of the Medical Committee. As time went on a valuable collection of these began to accumulate. Large scale models of various parts of the body were presented by some of the teachers and committee members. A life-size anatomical model, which could be taken to pieces and which showed the various regions of the body, superficial and deep, was purchased in Paris at the Auzoux laboratories, the cost being defrayed by Miss A.E.Keep, late Treasurer to the School.

The same donor also supplied a set of sectional bookcases to house the nucleus of a medical library. Many standard works of reference in general medicine and surgery, together with a representative collection of homoeopathic literature, were also added to help build up a good medical reference library.

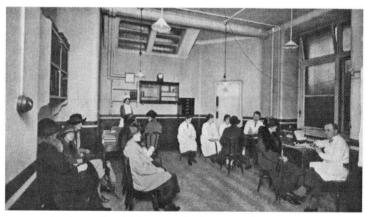

Students sit with Doctors in the Outpatients' Room

Practical Training
One of the first teaching improvements was the setting up of tutorial classes for instruction in physical diagnosis and related matters. This was the specific responsibility of Dr T.G.Stonham MD, a lecturer at the School and an assistant physician at the LHH. Practical experience

in all areas of medical practice was high on the agenda for each day. All students received a personal timetable allotting them to a particular teacher or clinic in the out-patient department, wards, daily dressings' room, or operating theatres.

In the out-patient clinics the students sat with the doctors to hear the patients' accounts of their ailments and the doctors' questions, to take part in the examination of the cases and to see and hear the treatment, and then to observe the progress of the patients at subsequent visits. The students were constantly encouraged to ask questions. As the hospital existed for the patients and not for the students, and as the out-patients' clinics were normally crowded and busy, if students failed to ask questions of the doctors at that time they would so easily have missed valuable opportunities.

A Former Student's Advice
Kathleen Singleton Fisher, a student of the 1914-15 session, wrote from the then Belgian Congo about this particular point of asking questions. She gave good advice to subsequent students:

> Learn every bit of practical work you can: bedmaking, blanket baths, douching, enemas, passing catheters, sterilizing, hot packs etc.

As regards small surgical operations and dressings, and such things as putting on splints she wrote,

> Learn to do these things yourselves. It is far better to pluck up courage and attempt these things first under the surgeon's eye. Fancy a busy mission doctor saying to you, 'Open that abscess' and then leaving you! If you've done it before you have far more self-confidence.
>
> I found at the MSM that I could learn to *do* just as much or little as I liked. I found it took a tremendous amount of courage to do anything, and I often held back when I might have taken opportunities of learning how to put into practice what I had learned theoretically.
>
> When I got out here I simply *had* to do things without help and often I wished I had not been so scared when at home.

Examinations
From the first, written examinations were conducted in most of the subjects and in some oral or practical. Prizes were awarded to the best students. Every endeavour was given to making these as useful as possible, consisting normally of medical books, surgical instruments,

or cases of medicines. The cost was usually met by friends of the School. Many of the lecturers awarded their own prizes, usually books.

It is possible that in the early days there was a tendency on the part of some of the lecturers to forget that they were talking to non-professional students. Time showed how difficult it was to select what was essential and practicable, but experience as usual eventually enabled the right level of instruction to be found. Synopses of the lectures were at one time provided in advance but this proved difficult to keep up and so was discontinued.

A Popular Subject

Dentistry became increasingly popular as the School developed. Instruction was at first given at certain local private clinics within the vicinity of the Hospital but as its own dental clinic grew under the oversight of Mr A.R.Stacey, so instruction for MSM students became an increasingly normal part of the routine. Both Mr Stacey and his colleague Mr Hill took a real interest in helping the students to gain a useful understanding of this subject, even to the extent of establishing an evening dental clinic in order to increase the teaching material.

The Tale of an Unusual Tooth

News soon began to come from many areas of the world, indicating how great an asset in missionary endeavour were the results of instruction in dentistry. Writing from Morocco, Miss **Agnes Hubbard** described something of this:

> In 1913 I took the dentistry course at the MSM. I had then been on the mission field for 20 years and so realized something of the terrible suffering that can come through bad teeth alone. The people here had only the help of the local barber and he has only one pair of forceps for the whole set of teeth! The tales one is told of how the barber drags the patient around his shop before he gets the offending tooth out - and very often only gets a part of it - are enough to make one feel cold.
>
> Since I took the dental course at the MSM I have never lacked for patients; last year I had 415 dental patients and this year (1919) it looks at present as though I shall have a good many more than that. The ladies here say that they like me to go to their homes because they can talk to me, and put off the evil hour while doing so! When the barber is summoned, then the patient's face must be covered, except the mouth, and the poor woman herself may not say a word. However, if the folks come to us, or if it is the better class folks who send for us to go to

them, it all makes openings for the message of the gospel we are here to give.

Being Moslems, of course, the people very much look down on Christians, and class them with the Jews and the dogs. A while ago I took out a tooth for a woman who was very pleased with me, and wished me every blessing of heaven, and kissed my head and hands. Then she picked up the tooth and said to it, 'Oh, you enemy! I will take you and pound you to powder for all the pain you have given me - you DOG! you JEW! you CHRISTIAN!'

She quite forgot that it was a Christian hand that had just removed the enemy from the native soil!

So I feel I owe a very great debt to the MSM and to the dentists, who had such patience with often clumsy students.

Publicity

As the School was an entirely professional institution and was not connected with any specific religious society or denomination, it was at first necessary to know how best to introduce it to the circles where it would be most useful. Without previous credentials this could be done only through the ordinary channels of advertisements. After a time, letters were addressed to, and interviews sought with the heads of the various missionary societies. On a few occasions the School sent exhibits illustrative of its equipment and teaching to large missionary exhibitions, such as The Orient Exhibition in London, and the exhibition held by the Baptist Missionary Society in St.George's Hall, Liverpool.

Decachords

An outstanding student of the 1913-14 session was Arthur Gladstone Clarke who later went on to serve for many years in North China with the Christian Mission to Many Lands. Arthur became an ardent student of the Homoeopathic Materia Medica and had considerable success in its use both for his own family, amongst his fellow missionaries and the many nationals amongst whom he worked.

He returned for his first furlough in 1923 and did a further term's study at MSM. Shortly after returning to China he published in 1925 a book entitled Decachords. This was a concise little book on the materia medica written particularly for lay missionaries involved with elementary medical work. Covering about 80 of the most commonly used remedies, each one was condensed under its 10 most salient characteristics. Later that year, on presenting this book to students, Dr

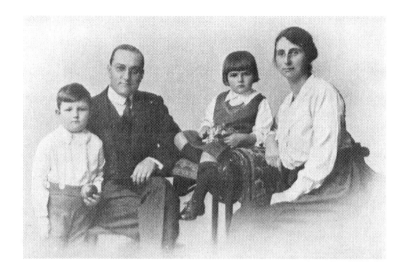

Mr. Gladstone Clarke and Family

Edwin Neatby was amused to find that some of them thought it was too elementary for their use! Little were they to know that it was to go through four editions and after the addition of 40 other remedies in more abbreviated form is still being sold by the MSM in the 21st century.

The Ethos of the Missionary School of Medicine

By the time the School came of age certain clear features were emerging which gave it its main ethos for most of the remaining century. Some of these may be listed here:

- Nearly all its teaching was carried out under one roof at the London Homoeopathic Hospital. Appendix A contains a brief synopsis of the Hospital, which contributed so greatly to the early development and subsequent work of the School, as acknowledged in the MSM Constitution.

- The School was non-residential except for a brief period during the second world war.

- In the various special departments the teaching has been mainly done by specialists in their respective fields.

- The fees have always been kept at as moderate a level as possible.

- Due to the generosity of various donors over the years, free Studentships have been made available to 'the most suitable applicants', determined by their financial needs and by their ability to profit from the training.

- Although the Council of the School has always kept its doors as widely open as possible, preference has been given to those specifically called to overseas missionary service.

- Students have been required to agree never to assume or accept the title of doctor or to practise in the United Kingdom.

- The Council always discouraged proselytism amongst the students, coming as they did from a wide variety of Christian denominations and international backgrounds.

The Constitution of 1951, to which passing reference is made later, clarified the Christian faith by stating:

> The benefits of the training courses shall be available to all persons otherwise eligible, provided always that their beliefs and teaching conform to those commonly associated with Protestant religion and no other person shall be eligible. The judgement in every case as to whether any person is, or is not, eligible shall rest with the Executive Committee. Should any difficulty arise in coming to a decision, the matter shall be referred to the Council.

3 Recognition And Scepticism

A Remarkable Fact

At the conclusion of the 1925-26 session it was recorded that 523 students had passed through the School since it began, the majority of whom were doing splendid service for the Lord all over the world and putting into practice the medical instruction they had received, as a major tool in their work of evangelism. By this time the School had become well established as a recognized training institution in medicine and surgery for non-medical missionaries. Situated as it was in the heart of London, next door to the world-famous Hospital for Sick Children in Great Ormond Street and where several great medical training hospitals had long been established, it was quite remarkable that this rather unique School was recognized by all the rest.

Few of its students were university graduates and most had limited academic qualifications. Yet each day these students were receiving instruction from some of the best qualified specialists available in their respective medical and surgical fields.

There was an interesting note in the July edition that year of *The International Review of Missions* about the medical work of non-medical missionaries. It praised their willingness, adaptability and professional skill to render physical aid which was often thrust upon them. The author, Dr Lerrigo wrote, *'It is wholly impossible to record all the worthwhile services of this nature'*, and it is worth noting that he went on to suggest that *'a special medical treatise for use by non-medical missionaries is needed'*. We have already recorded how the MSM foresaw this need and remedied it by publishing its own Manual of Tropical Medicine and Hygiene for Missionaries, compiled by Drs E.A. and T.M.Neatby.

Two New Features

There was a larger proportion of students staying for the complete three-term course and there was a good prospect for the 1927-28 session. Dr Edwin Neatby, the Honorary Secretary (later to be known as The Dean), reported that the School had just *'experienced for the first time a whole session in its new **lecture room'**. He went on to mention the distinct advantages of this new facility, although for some reason there was no telephone in the Secretary's office. Apparently the difficulty was not in getting the telephone, but arranging for somebody to answer it!

At the Annual Meeting it was announced that, *'a new prize* had been *given by some anonymous friends in memory of Dr John Clarke, to the best MSM student of the year'*. In subsequent years it was a much sought after honour to be worthy of the title, 'Clarke Prizeman of the Year'.

A Knighthood for the Honorary Treasurer
A further enhancement to the reputation of the Missionary School of Medicine came when its Honorary Treasurer, Dr John Weir, received a knighthood from the King (KCVO).

A Full House
As the years passed the popularity and acceptance of the training given at the School was particularly indicated by the comparatively high numbers of candidates requesting admittance to the courses being offered. 36 applied for the 25th Jubilee Session, of which 24 were women. In the 1928-29 year, 32 students did the course, representing twelve missionary societies around the world. Even during the early thirties, when the United Kingdom experienced severe industrial problems arising out of the General Strike, 23 registered for the twenty-seventh session (1930-31). A very important factor in the recognition and success of the School was the generous hospitality of the LHH which from the first opened its doors, wards and clinics to the students, furnishing them all with such knowledge and experience as enabled them to look after their own lives in a hostile environment and to assist them look after the lives of their fellow missionaries, and in doing such practical remedial ministrations as were called for amongst the people where they lived. The work of the School was carried on with characteristic skill, kindness and keenness by members of the Hospital's medical and surgical staff - and even from the porters - so that the students received a training and opportunities second to none in efficiency and value.

So much of the remarkable growth and success since its inception was particularly due to the work of the School's Dean, Dr E.A.Neatby. He worked unceasingly, giving a great deal of his time and strength and personal supervision to its daily well-being. His enthusiasm kept the School going especially when its friends were few and its prospects dim.   His professional skill was always freely given;   his wisdom shaped its form and its course. It was not too much to record that the Missionary School of Medicine became an enduring memorial to him.

Rumbles of Dissent

Under God, such was the blessing that was being achieved through the training being provided that some missionary societies were showing signs of scepticism about its teaching of homoeopathy, and the prominence it was giving to medical training at the expense of time for spiritual development.

Regarding the first of these criticisms, it would be fair to say that at different times throughout the life of the School objections from a variety of sources were aimed at homoeopathy, discrediting the emphasis given to this subject. It must be remembered however, that the venue for the School throughout its long life was the London Homoeopathic Hospital.   Many of their professional staff were the students' constant lecturers and they were always keen to support the efficacy of that branch of medicine, as we shall note from time to time.

Beyond that, throughout the School's history reports were received and made public of the way in which missionaries who trained at the MSM found homoeopathy to be so effective in their treatment of disease.

Speaking at one of the Annual Meetings of the School, the Dean said this:

> I want to say just one word about the position of homoeopathy at this School. We have the great privilege of working at this Hospital but there are quite a lot of people who keep away from us because we teach homoeopathy, and we are not a bit ashamed of it. It is one of the very grandest assets that we have.   We teach everything else that other schools teach, and all the resources of the medical sciences are at our command, and those who study here go out wonderfully well equipped, quite apart from homoeopathy. *The position of homoeopathy in this School is that it is an addendum to all that is taught in other schools that have the same objects as ourselves.*

Writing from Upper Burma, the Revd **Timothy Houghton** MA, who later served as   President of the School for almost thirty years said:

> I can never be too thankful for my year's course at the MSM in 1923-24. I went with the intention of getting all the good out of the course, while studiously avoiding anything to do with homoeopathy,

but my interest was soon aroused and I felt that I had come, not to a colony of cranks but to people who really knew what they were talking about. As I watched in the clinics, I was amazed at some of the successes.

But I have been very much more amazed by the successes I myself have experienced out here! I should not have thought it possible that a complete amateur like myself could prove so useful. I am able to stop attacks of dengue fever with Eupatorium Perfoliatum as soon as I begin to feel the prodrome. This is a great relief as during two rainy seasons I have had four attacks of dengue, which all pretty well laid me out and wasted a lot of time.

Timothy Houghton went on to describe some other cases which he was able to treat successfully, using homoeopathy. One was a man who travelled 90 miles for treatment for chronic pain in one leg and thigh, after having had treatment in his local hospital. Causticum was prescribed and when he reported back in a month's time he walked into the dispensary himself. Previously, he had crawled and could not stand. He was most indignant when asked if he *really* felt better, and said he could walk with ease and was now able to carry on his trade.

Another woman, with terrible burning pains in her chest looked seriously ill, and herself was quite sure she was going to die, was treated with Arsenicum Album 30. She said she had already had about 40 different medicines and only came to the dispensary as a last resort. After a sharp aggravation at about 1 a.m. she recovered, and for the first time for months felt really well!

Timothy concludes,

Of course, I regard this all as a means to an end, the evangelisation of these dear people ... every intending missionary student should go to the MSM!

Another striking testimony to the validity of homoeopathy came from **Mrs Vollrath** who had been one of the earliest students in 1907-08. When working with her husband in Turkestan they were returning to their base in Thuringia, a journey lasting many months. At one stop, they met with a great epidemic of typhus. Their stock of homoeopathic drugs coming to an end, they did not know what to do. Her husband prepared some Pyrogenium homoeopathically and the results of it were so striking, that, given at the beginning of the illness many patients recovered rapidly.

On arriving at the town of Omsk they were forced to remain on the train for a week. The stations were indescribable.... 'One train after another came in with people suffering from dysentery, cholera, typhus, smallpox and all kinds of diseases, and little was being done by the authorities to contain these diseases.'

She and her sister then became very ill themselves with cholera. The memory of the lectures she was given at the MSM about cholera then came back to her - severe cramps, loss of muscle control. She began to squint and lose her voice - the feeling of a channel going through her head from one ear to the other, 'I shall never forget'.

They had some Camphor with them and used it a little, which brought them some relief but they thought they would die. Meanwhile her husband had been looking for some Arsenicum Album which they had carried with them, but had lost when they were forced to leave the train. On the sixth day it was found and after just two doses, the vomiting ceased altogether and they began to recover.

When the doctor came along for his usual visit (they had by then been taken to a military hospital) he asked, 'Whatever have you done?' When told, he shook his head and could not believe it. In her letter Mrs Vollrath continued, 'Near our ward (*you* would have called it a stable) the people were lying about with dysentery, crying with pain day and night. One of the field surgeons asked my husband if he had a remedy for these sufferers. "Oh yes", he replied, "I would give Mercurius Corrosivus." They went to the dispensary together and my husband told him how to prepare it and when it was administered the patients recovered quickly.

'The field surgeon took it to his other patients in the district and found the same results. He was dumbfounded and said, "I have never heard of this new treatment and I would like to learn more about it having seen the marvellous results." We gave him some instructions, as much as we were able to, and he was learning eagerly and taking down notes.'

Growing in Grace
The second cause for scepticism was what was seen as a lack of time spent on spiritual development in favour of medical instruction. Quoting from a page of the annual report for the 1926-27 session on Spiritual Values this matter is mentioned as follows:

> It will be specially gratifying to those in whose hearts the evangelistic and spiritual side of a missionary's work ranks easily first, to know that while in training at this School the students are encouraged to hold meetings to maintain their spiritual tone. For many years this

has been regularly done. In the privacy of our own lecture room, prayer, praise and Bible meetings are held.

In some missionary circles it has been feared that a missionary so trained might be liable to the temptation to give up a very large proportion of time to medical study to the detriment of his or her primary function.

It is of course, impossible to state that this never happened but we have repeated assurances that the removal of prejudice, and the gaining of confidence in medical work made for opportunities of a spiritual nature which otherwise could not have been possible.

The results the School were able to publish could not have been obtained without dedicated training, and it is conspicuous how constantly prayer for guidance and blessing accompanied the practice of the students. *It seems certain that the spiritual value of the training entirely outweighed the possibility of over-zeal in its use.*

The Museum receives a unique specimen

During the 1928-29 session the gift of an epidiascope by a Mrs A. Lloyd was much appreciated, and the same year the Museum also received *a very interesting and sentimental addition.* When the renowned missionary and explorer, Dr David Livingstone's body was brought home to this country in 1874 it needed to be specifically identified. It was remembered that Livingstone's left arm had been broken by a lion in the early years of his work in Africa. That fracture never united and he was left with a fracture of the left humerus which was permanently impaired.

It was thought that if this fracture could be recognized it would serve, with other facts that were known, as an identification of his body. At that time Dr E.B.Roche, a long supporter of the School, who was a friend of Dr Neatby, was assisting Sir William Ferguson, to remove the bone from the arm and identify it. A cast was then taken of the bone - the only cast taken - and this was eventually presented to the Museum by Mrs Roche. It was a unique exhibit and the School was proud to possess it.

An Unusual Comment

Dr Edwin Neatby was a person of considerable originality. On one occasion he said:

'The Missionary School of Medicine was *unsectarian* in its position - medically, professionally, and from the religious standpoint.'
He then went on to introduce another word which he had recently come across, which struck him as very interesting and appropriate:

'The School was not only unsectarian but *insectarian*. Insects conveyed a large number of diseases, especially tropical diseases: they were carriers of various poisons and germs; flies, fleas bugs, lice, mosquitos and sandflies, all played their part. In the Museum at 2 Powis Place drawings could be seen of all, or most, of these insects, together with actual specimens, carefully prepared and preserved for teaching purposes.'

Most of the MSM students were able to explain something of these various carriers of disease. Many of them, having completed their course, would rank as heroes and heroines as they proceeded abroad to face odds which they would not have been called upon to face if they had remained in this country. The most ordinary Christian person, when filled by the Holy Spirit, and trained at the MSM was wonderfully equipped to face enormous odds, as many letters have demonstrated.

Losses and Gains
To celebrate and mark the thirtieth anniverary of the founding of the School a fund was launched called 'The Thirty Year Fund' and an appeal made for an initial sum of two thousand pounds (a lot of money in those far-off times). It was launched with spectacular enthusiasm and hope by the Council of the School and soon money began to pour in, in large and small amounts, every contribution being acknowledged in the printed Annual Report, circulated worldwide to past students and numerous supporters. Sadly however, the following year (1933-34), this celebratory fund became a Memorial Fund to mark the sudden passing into the Lord's presence of the two leading members of the School.

The Dean, Dr Edwin Awdas Neatby, had been a key figure right from the start. The President, Dr Stuart Holden, among several others, paid a glowing tribute to him:

> It is no exaggeration to say that the School largely owed its existence to Dr Neatby's interest, enthusiasm and constant hard work. None who have come in contact with him have doubted that he made the School what it is, and that, in losing him, we lose our guide and counsellor, our chief and captain, our inspiration and our mainstay.

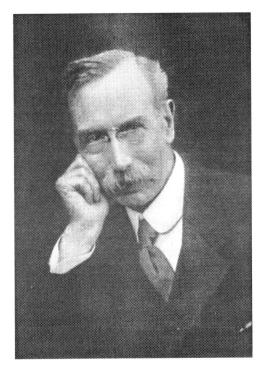

Dr. Neatby, Honorary Secretary

All through his life he earned by his uprightness and complete integrity, the respect and admiration of those who met him, but in addition, he had the winning ways of a man without any self-seeking or personal vanity, and so attracted not only respect but love.

With every year of his leadership there was increased efficiency and to work under him or with him was both a privilege and a joy. The School itself is his best memorial, and all who give thanks for his life have an obligation placed upon them by their very recognition of what the School owes to him, to ensure that it continues even more fully than was possible under his leadership.

Dr Neatby's widow accepted a seat on the Council and the fact that she was still associated with the School was a great satisfaction to everyone.

The blow that fell near the beginning of that year in the death of the Dean, was added to at the end of the year by the unexpected death of its President, the Revd Dr Stuart Holden. Amid all his many activities and the many claims on his time and energy, he always kept a place for the Missionary School of Medicine. He was preparing to give all that he could to fill the vacancy left by Dr Neatby's passing, when he too was summoned into the presence of the Lord, whom he served so faithfully and well.

He had been Vicar of St Paul's Church, Portman Square in London and was widely known in this country and in America as a winsome preacher. He was Honorary Home Director of the great China Inland Mission, founded by Hudson Taylor, a post which gave him an intimate acquaintance with missionary candidates, and he was always a strong believer in the necessity of giving such personnel training in the elements of medicine and surgery. Now his loss was keenly felt by all associated with him in the work of directing the MSM and his passing left a gap difficult to fill.

A story worth noting was recounted by Dr Holden on his last visit to the School.   He had heard of a minister who moved to a new living. Having installed an electric bell on the front door of his house, when he moved to his new house he took out the battery from the bell, disconnected the wires and carried the bell and fittings away with him. On arrival he found a doorbell already in place and his bell was not needed.   However, thinking that he would make such use as he could of the old one, he turned it into a lamp for the sidetable by his desk. He bought all that was needed and fixed it up to the battery, and turned on the switch, but nothing happened. He was greatly disappointed and called an electrician to look into it.

This young man at once said, 'Surely you know it takes far more elctricity to keep a lamp shining than to ring a bell: it takes very little power to make a noise, but a good deal more to make a light!'

Dr Holden then went on to say - in what were virtually his last words to the students - that students of the MSM had to be lights and not mere noise makers. Their preaching would never be authenticated unless their lives gave it strength and power. As they went out from the *commencement* provided at the MSM they should pray that the fellowship of the Spirit of God might be a real force in their experience so that they might become a means of extending the Kingdom of God. He prayed that the blessing of the Holy Spirit might be upon their future labours.

Miss Goodin, the School's Secretary, also retired at the end of this 31st session after many years of dedicated service. The School Monitor for the year, Brian Forbes, said about her leaving, 'It is with deep regret that we learn we are to be the last of her *'children'* to be under the loving and maternal care of our Secretary.' Her duties were taken over by Miss Elizabeth J.Bargh SRN, MCSP, who already had years of experience as a teacher of nurses. She was to remain in this post - eventually upgraded to Warden - for the next 31 years!

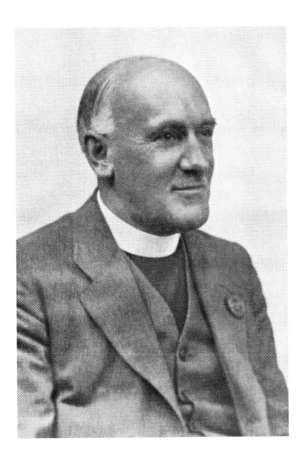

Rev. W. H. Aldis, President

Another gain the School experienced at that time was the appointment of the Revd W.H.Aldis to succed Dr Stuart Holden as President. At the time Mr Aldis was the Home Director of the China Inland Mission, and when asked by the Council of the School to assume this post, he accepted the offer with some diffidence. Writing about his appointment, he said:

It was my privilege to know the late Dean of the School and I had a little insight into the devotion with which he gave himself to the work and what a joy it was for him to know that through this agency he was making a valuable contribution to the great work of world evangelization. It has also been my privilege to have had a close association with the late president of the School, who took such a warm personal interest in its work and who by voice and pen sought to further its interests. Therefore, it is with a feeling that I am entering into a great succession that I associate myself with the School, and if I am able to do anything to extend its influence I shall be profoundly thankful.

Mr. Aldis served for many years as a missionary in China and so was well suited to the task presented to him in this new capacity.

During the session 1933-34 much work of a spiritual nature was undertaken by the students in spite of their smaller numbers. There was a ministry of song in the wards nearly every Sunday evening and open-air meetings were held in the neighbourhood around the LHH especially targeting the children.

It was the constant effort of the Council of the School that kept the teaching up-to-date. From time to time, because of the pressure of other commitments, lecturers had to resign, but usually younger men and women were good enough to step into the breach and most of the formal lectures were given by experts in their different fields, (Appendix B). Visual aids and models were extensively used in instruction to ensure greater clarity and understanding.

A Suggestion Blossoms
It was the Rev Stanley Franklin, a student of the 1912-13 session, a Congregationalist, who served for some years in South America with EUSA, who first suggested the formation of a body which eventually developed into the Students' Fellowship. He urged the publication of an occasional medical magazine for circulation among former students with the idea of keeping them in touch with one another, and to disseminate new items of medical or surgical knowledge likely to be of service to them. To add to the varied ups and downs of the 31st session was the actual launching of the The Students' Fellowship which was to feature prominently in the following years. This also was instituted in memory of the late Dean and initially was under the joint leadership of Miss Evelyn Saunders and the Revd Noel Clarke. It aimed to link up all students, past and present in mutual friendship, and to give

assistance where necessary to those working abroad. An annual Fellowship Day was inaugurated, when students on home leave and those working in the UK, as well as interested friends, were welcomed.

The first event of this kind was held in May 1935 and took the form of an afternoon lecture on, Homoeopathy and the Missionary, given by Dr P.G.Quinton, one of the regular teaching staff of the School. After the lecture, visits were arranged to various hospital departments and the Tropical Museum in the School, following which tea was served. In the evening, a devotional meeting was held - students gave their contribution in song - and the School chorus 'Unafraid' was heartily rendered! Mr D.M.Miller of the Africa Inland Mission gave a powerful message on the Significance of the Cross. Many friendships were made and renewed, and no one could have failed to be re-inspired for further service.

A bi-annual magazine was to be issued and sent to all members. Also a Bureau was established through which members working overseas could procure drugs, medical and surgical supplies, and receive professional advice in the treatment of difficult cases. Through the Students' Fellowship its members contributed financially to the work of MSM as half of each subscription was given directly to it. During its first year 700 former students were circulated with information concerning its establishment and 80 members paid the annual subscription of five shillings.

Growth of the Students' Fellowship
After experiencing some teething problems, the Students' Fellowship developed well and much of this was due to its Secretary Mr G.F.Price and his assistant Miss Harper, both of whom gave of their time and interest unstintingly. The Drug Bureau was very active and correspondence to do with enquiries from past students seeking professional help concerning difficult cases came in from all over the world.

More Losses
One of the problems facing the writing of this history is the inevitable fact of human frailty. Spanning as it does a complete century, we recall the almost immortal words of that great Victorian poet, Alfred Lord Tennyson, who when writing about 'The Brook,' said:
> '...For men may come and men may go but I go on forever.'

During the session of 1936-37 the School again suffered severe losses through death, in particular, that of Dr **George Burford** who had been associated with the MSM since its inception; in fact it was he who first suggested the idea back in 1903, although his great friend and colleague, the late Dean, was responsible for its early development. On one occasion, when proposing a vote of thanks at one of the Annual Meetings of the School, Dr Burford said:

> He wished to make one reference to China. He had had the good fortune to have been there for sometime, where he had the privilege to have met one of the most distinguished medical men of the age, Professor Manson, and had the opportunity of working with him.
>
> On one occasion they were called to see a young lady, the wife of a Mandarin, who had given birth to a baby. She was so ill that when they saw her they realized that absolutely nothing could be done. Yet, had she been seen earlier, any student of the MSM after only a few month's training could have saved her. 19 days of agony had been endured by this lady of birth and breeding, who was absolutely devoid of any assistance such as could have been given by a student of the School.

Dr Burford went on to say,

> **It was very desirable to spread the practice of medical missionaries, qualified to bring ease to the body in healing, as an introduction to the Christian Faith. The work done in this particular institution was of great value; it was the most striking instance of the association of homoeopathy and the religion taught by Christ.**

Dr Burford did not know of any similar institution in any other part of the world where these two revolutionary doctrines were so satisfactorily welded.

Another great loss at the same time was that of Mr Stacey who lectured so long in dentistry. 'It is hard to imagine the School without Mr Stacey, who was unfailing in his support and tireless in his work for us', wrote Dr C.E.Wheeler, a member of the Council.

Financial Matters
At a time of immense financial difficulty, owing largely to the national economic recession of the early thirties, the outstanding financial event of the 1930-31 session - was a large gift by a generous donor in memory of her sister who had been an old friend of the School. This gift came most opportunely as it enabled certain important and needful purchases and alterations to be made, for which the normal income

would have been unequal. How often the School was to experience the gracious provision of the Lord for such emergency needs.

However, the problems of running such a voluntary organization as the Missionary School of Medicine during a time of national financial crisis was brought to the attention of its supporters by the printing *on red paper* of a special leaflet for insertion in the annual report for the following session which was distributed all over the world. It read:

> The Honorary Auditor, T. Burton Miller, Esq., C.A., has warned the Council that the reserve funds of the School have recently been so considerably reduced that new subscribers are essential to its success. Unless increased income can be secured there is serious danger that the School may be seriously crippled, or entirely unable to carry on its worldwide beneficent work...

The fact that the MSM continued for another seventy years, although now with a different method of achieving its objectives, must indicate both God's gracious provision and the generosity of his people.

Every Penny Helps

An urgent appeal was made during that session for the replacement of essential equipment in order to bring it up to date. Dr Daukes of the Wellcome Bureau of Scientific Research inspected the School's own Museum and made recommendations for its improvement. As a result, a list of some of the needs was circulated to supporters.

The prices quoted reveal just how much the value of money has changed when compared with the present day. A large gift of one thousand pounds in securities was donated during the year and 119 people subscribed to the general fund. Gifts ranged from £100 to half a crown (12½ pence). Every subscriber's name was printed in the Annual Report together with the amount given! The income that year was £782.18s.4d.

An Appreciation from Northern India

An encouraging letter came that year from Mr **Len Moules** serving in Northern India with the Worldwide Evangelisation Crusade of which he was later to become General Secretary. He had recently arrived there having completed the MSM course the previous year. He wrote:

> Ever since my arrival out here I have been thrust into medical work of one type or another. In only two months, over 2,000 patients passed

through our hands. I cannot praise God enough for the great value of the MSM course. Through the knowledge imparted to me, the great closed doors of Nepal opened on four occasions to allow me to enter to treat sick men and women. This not only afforded opportunity for practice but it allowed the glorious Gospel to be left by the spoken and printed word. Minor surgery under very doubtful conditions has been attempted and teeth extractions have been so numerous as to have lost their novelty.

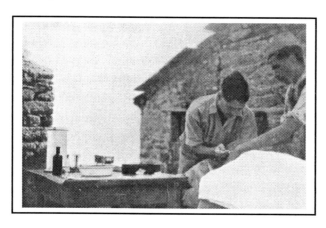

A Cataract Operation, the Tibetan Border
From Mr. Len Moules

During my stay in the plains, about 30 people left our dispensary with a good measure of sight restored by means of cataract operations. Doctor wants me to get proficient and has given me further instruction. We do not use the 'needling' method but do Smith's intrecapsular extraction. I have assisted with about sixteen cases and done three myself. I shall be writing to the Students' Fellowship Bureau for a cataract set before I go off to the Tibetan border next year.

Cases of leprosy and venereal disease have been satisfactorily treated but if there is anything which has given me pleasure it was the immediate response of two Indian women suffering from pneumonia when treated with Bryonia and Phosphorus, and a case of malaria which had a great recovery by doses of Natrum Muriaticum.

How inadequate the above items sound when compared with the amount and variety of the work, but how thankful I am to have been allowed to have had such tuition as that given at the MSM. Praise God for the School and for those School days.

A Salesperson for the MSM

In the years immediately prior to the Second World War, the Council felt that it would greatly enhance the reputation of the School, and make its work more widely known, if someone could travel about the country and address meetings in colleges and churches on behalf of the School. Hence it was a great delight when Mrs Douglas Porter was appointed for this ministry. Sadly, nothing is recorded about the effectiveness of her assignment.

Real Dedication

The session held during 1938-39 was one of the best in the School's history with 28 students, and it was of particular interest that nine out of that number were missionaries on furlough, proving the *need* as well as the *value* of the course: they were commended for giving up nine months of their home leave in order to study at the School.

As this session drew towards its close it became increasingly obvious that political tensions, especially in Europe, were moving towards a climax. This happened at the beginning of September 1939 when the German Chancellor, Adolf Hitler, against all his promises to the contrary, invaded Poland. Britain declared war on Germany on Sunday September 3rd, an action which greatly altered the course of history and changed most peoples' lives; not least being the well ordered routine and running of the Missionary School of Medicine.

4 The School Beats The Blitz
(The War Years 1939 - 1945)

Words of Warning

> We are at the beginning of a conflict which may be of long duration. The war has been precipitated by one man, who, to gratify his own personal ambitions for world domination, is ready to break his most solemn pledges and to inflict upon mankind the most fearful carnage the world has known. Such callous inhumanity, which has already been evidenced in the relentless persecution of the Jews of Germany, and the torture of loyal pastors in prison and concentration camps, is a menace to the whole world. For this reason all lovers of liberty, justice and truth, simply must take a stand against this evil thing. *That is why we are at war.*

So wrote the President of the Missionary School of Medicine, the Revd W.H.Aldis, in the Forward of the Annual Report for 1939. He went on to write:

> But war will not end these evil things, for they originate in the unregenerate heart of man. There is only one real remedy and that is the gospel of the Lord Jesus Christ, and the greatest contribution that can be made towards meeting the deepest need of the world is the proclamation of that gospel, which is 'the power of God unto salvation to everyone that believeth' (Roman 1:16).
>
> The Missionary School of Medicine is doing its part to further the work of evangelization, by seeking to give to the missionaries of the gospel, the further equipment of a useful measure of medical and surgical knowledge, which so often has proved to be the first step in opening hearts to receive the message of salvation.
>
> The report of the year has to be abbreviated in order to economize, (paper was one of the first things to be rationed) but the School hopes to carry on its work through the days of the war.

Boarding Accommodation

Early on in the war, the London Homoeopathic Hospital kindly arranged for a number of male students to live in the house at No.3 Powis Place, adjoining the School.

Consequently, an appeal was sent out to the supporters which read as follows:

> In these difficult days of rising prices, and war conditions, the planning of a menu is no easy task, especially when expenditure must be kept within the limits of the purses of missionary students. Gifts in kind,

however small, would be most gratefully received. Such contributions as flour, oatmeal, rice, barley, canned or fresh fruit and other edible goods - which can be spared - will be welcomed. Flowers and plants would also be much appreciated to brighten the School and the students' house. Will kind friends please send all gifts direct to the Secretary who will gladly acknowledge them.

Trenches in Queen's Square
The first session under wartime conditions in 1939 started with 15 students and inevitably the course suffered limitations due to the exingencies of war but every effort was made to keep these to a minimum. Trenches were dug in Queen's Square adjoining the Hospital and students were obliged to attend Air Raid Precaution (ARP) lectures. Later in the year, more students came for part of the course, including several missionaries who were on furlough. Dr Ernest Muir of the British Empire Leprosy Relief Association gave lectures on that disease and an invitation was extended to students from other missionary training colleges, of which 30 accepted and attended the lectures.

Various lay people helped the School in a voluntary and useful capacity throughout the year including Miss Tester, a past student, who spent 2 or 3 days each week rearranging the Museum exhibits; Mr Hamilton, a handyman, also helped in the Museum doing all the carpentry work gratuitously, as well as other odd jobs about the School including photography. The MSM was also fortunate in securing the help of another former student, Miss Sibley, for clerical help - she had spent some time in the Belgian Congo but had to return for health reasons.

A Year of Anxiety
1940 was a year of anxiety for all those connected with the running of the School but, in the goodness of God, its work and ministry was able to continue. Twenty-two students registered for training, but their safety while travelling in the heart of the Capital as it was subjected to much heavy bombing, plus their safety when at the School was always a matter of deep concern, daily threatening the School's very life. Changes at the LHH through evacuation and depletion of staff were also a challenge. The Council were encouraged by the Word of the Lord which came to them in power, to bring comfort and wisdom. *'Be still and know that I am God'*, and so God's plan for the session gradually unfolded. It was somewhat ironic that the doctors, having

less private work, were able and willing to give more detailed teaching. Gradually the clinical work increased and students had the privilege of attending other institutions. The Bermondsey Medical Mission and the Lansdowne Medical Mission admitted the students to their dental clinics. The Poplar Hospital for Accidents also opened its doors, thus meeting an urgent need, as in the nature of things casualty work and minor operations were this hospital's outstanding feature, giving MSM students the opportunity of seeing and carrying out such surgical treatments as they would later be called upon to undertake when abroad on active missionary service.

Another limitation the School faced owing to the war was the closing of the Hospital for Tropical Diseases, but resulting from the kind interest and concern of Dr W.E.Cooke - by that time a Council member - students were received for clinical instruction at the Seamen's Hospital, Greenwich, where Dr Wingfield demonstrated and emphasized such points as missionaries were liable to encounter in tropical work. The Welcome Museum was also closed but the Malarial Control Course was arranged, as in previous years, at the Ross Institute and the students attended this with great benefit.

Hence, by such means, the examination standard was well maintained for the year. One student in particular, Ronald Male, who was later to write *The Bible & Homoeopathy*, a graduate of the Auckland Bible Institute in New Zealand and an accepted candidate of the Central Asian Mission, showed very marked all-round ability. Three other students gained special merit.

The School management also inaugurated two new departures with the aim of developing the practical application of the course. The candidates entered for and successfully passed the British Red Cross Society's First Aid Examination and some trainees passed the advanced tests. A practical nursing examination was also conducted by Miss Andros, the matron of the LHH after Sister Barnes had given practical lectures. Miss Swaine, an experienced nurse examiner, also held a bandaging contest.

Student War Workers
No.3 Powis Place continued as a temporary hostel for ten male students and was 'a great convenience'. A suitable housekeeper, Mrs Hamilton, was 'at hand' to look after the welfare of those accommodated, all of whom paid rent to the LHH. Many kind friends responded to the Secretary's appeal in the previous year for contributions to the ever dwindling storecupboard!

On the more positive side, the students so housed became war-workers qualifying for all kinds of emergency assistance, and as the air raids increased throughout the autumn, they played a gallant part regardless of all risks and difficulties, earning the warmest praise of the civic authorities. Mr Charles Tett was awarded the George Medal for conspicuous bravery. He, together with five colleagues, saved the premises of the MSM from incendiary bombs. The official announcement was published in 'The London Gazette' as follows,

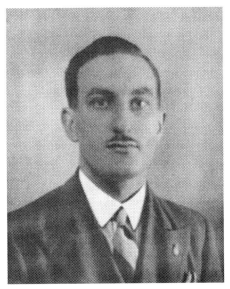

Mr. C.R.Tett, GM

When in a street during an enemy air-raid, Mr Tett heard the sound of a bomb descending. He dived for shelter under the wall of a public-house on the corner, at the same time pushing down two ladies who were near him. The impact followed almost immediately, and the blast caught him, severely shaking him. As the debris was falling he pushed an attache case over the ladies' heads to protect them.

Although dazed, Tett immediately attended as best he could to a number of severely injured persons in the vicinity. He then boarded a badly damaged bus and removed passengers who were injured and applied first-aid to the most seriously wounded. Throughout he showed great presence of mind and devotion to duty.

On another occasion when the Hospital was struck by an enemy bomb, Tett, with no thought for his own safety and on his own initiative, accompanied a stoker in crawling into the boiler house and over the boilers, to assist in shutting down the fire and cutting off the steam, an act requiring courage and resource of the highest order.

When congratulated on his conduct, Charles Tett showed an exemplary Christian spirit and merely said, 'I was glad to be in the place of such need'. Charles was from Weymouth and had previously trained at All Nations' Bible College where he received a first-class diploma. At the MSM also he won several first places for theoretical and practical medical work. He was waiting to go to Nigeria with the Sudan United Mission. Later, he spent many outstanding years of missionary service with the Church Mission Society in Kenya.

At the same time, the following awards were made by His Majesty the King to members of the staff of the LHH:
    The George Medal to Chief Engineer S.R. Campbell-Lyttle
    The George Medal to Night Porter F.C. Collins
    The British Empire Medal to Stoker R. Phillips.

Little information is available for 1941 but the work of the School went on with dedication from staff and students during those very difficult times. The President, Rev.W.H.Aldis, the following year expressed the conviction that God had undoubtedly led the Council to keep the doors of the School open, and though there might have been the temptation to close them in the face of national needs, the action had been fully justified. He and the Council thanked God for a government which appreciated spiritual values and permitted missionary students to continue their training.
    Sadly during the year the School suffered the loss through death of a number of staunch friends and helpers. Three Vice-presidents had passed away - Sir George Truscott, Sir Henry Davenport and the Revd Dr J.D.Jones. Mr Frank Piper, who had been a Council member since the earliest days also died. The Rt Revd Frank Houghton, the General Director of the China Inland Mission, became a Vice-president in that year (1942).

Looking Ahead
Although there were still three years to pass before the War was to end, already many people were thinking about and planning for post-war deveplopment. The Missionary School of Medicine was also anticipating advance and extension for its work, believing that there would then be a great need and demand for many well-equipped missionaries to go forth everywhere to 'preach and heal'.

During this year (1942-43) 15 students received training, attending the many and varied clinics. The ward sisters too continued to give instruction in all nursing procedures. On the financial side two factors greatly helped. The Hahnemann Trustees halved the rent on No 2, and the honorary Treasurer received three large donations amounting to £300 to meet current expenditure.

The year also saw the School completing 40 years of its work, and already several hundred men and women had gone from its doors to 'touch the ends of the earth' with the gospel. But all this was as 'a drop in the bucket' alongside the work and influence that was needed. Thousands of places in lands distant and also not so distant, so much needed the help which the School could provide, and however hard the years ahead might prove to be, it would have been a tragedy if the MSM had failed to extend its work. Thus, the Council were planning for *'a central building big enough to house its many activities in order to increase the student body'*.

The Fortieth Year

In spite of the complexities of the war situation, the 40th year saw a successful session. A new opening for eye work was given as the Royal Westminster Ophthalmic Hospital permitted MSM students to attend its clinics. In all countries cases of eye disease form a very large percentage of patients which students are called upon to help and although instruction was given at the Eye Clinic of the LHH, this further opportunity of seeing eye diseases in such a specialist hospital was invaluable.

Attendance at the Foot Clinic, particularly by those candidates expecting to major on itinerant walking evangelism, received greater attention, and the expert instruction given by Mr Le Rossignal was greatly valued.

The Students' Fellowship's Progress

All through the war years, the Students' Fellowship continued its activities due largely to the enthusiasm of its secretary, Mr G.J.P.Price and his assistant Miss B.P.Harper. Some frustration though, was noticeable on the leaders' part due to the failure of several ex-students to enrol as members. On the Annual Fellowship Day in 1943 an announcement was made which showed that the Fellowship was starting a fund through which books and medical outfits could be sent to those ex-students at work around the world.

The monthly meeting held by the Fellowship and known as 'The Prayer Circle' continued to be times of real spiritual uplift and refreshment. *'To look back with gratitude is much; to look forward with faith is more, and the Students' Fellowship ensures both'* was how the Secretary concluded his contribution to the Annual Report for that year.

Flying Bomb Attacks
Around the premises of the MSM in Powis Place much damage was sustained because of the vigorous attacks of the German airforce using its 'secret weapon', the 'Flying Bomb' which was a pilotless plane filled with high explosive which dived to earth when its fuel ran out. This was particularly intense during the 1944-45 session but the School itself was protected, without damage, and with no hindrance to its activities. Twenty-one students received training that year: 13 did the full course and the rest were part-time; most students were prospective missionary candidates but some were making use of a lengthened furlough due to the war, to obtain extra medical experience. The general shortage of doctors - so many were serving in the armed forces - threw extra burdens on the remaining medical staff of the LHH but however pressed, they never stinted in giving the MSM the best of their services. They helped, as always with that cheerful readiness which doubled the value of their teaching.

Bravely Coping with War-time Conditions
Whilst every subject in the syllabus was important and of the greatest value, certain lines were inevitably of greater importance than others. Tropical Diseases and Hygiene are subjects which all missionaries meet in one form or another and the School was blessed at that time to have Dr Cooke and Dr Gregg to give such important instruction. These lectures were supplemented by clinical tutorials at the Seamen's Hospital at Greenwich by Dr Wingfield, another expert in Tropical Medicine. Also during this session Professor Leiper extended to the students the privilege of a series of demonstrations in tropical parasitology in the London School of Tropical Hygiene.

All the normal features of teaching and practical opportunities which by now were a normal feature of MSM training continued in spite of war-time restrictions. Especially valued were the Compton-Burnett and the Honyman-Gillespie lectures on homoeopathy.

Several of the male students continued to be accommodated at No.3 Powis Place by arrangement with the LHH in return for certain war services in protecting the Hospital from enemy attack from the constant air-raids. This proved a very satisfactory arrangement for all those concerned.

Two foremost supporters of the School died during the year: Mr.E. Clifton-Brown, one of the Vice-presidents, and Dr T.Miller Neatby, cousin of the former Dean, who was a valued lecturer and friend of the many intakes of students for over 35 years. The help they each gave was incalculable and their loss immeasurable.

The Annual Meeting of the year which took place on June 30th was held as usual in the Examination Hall at Queen's Square accompanied by the noises of war. Air-raid alerts by sirens could be heard throughout most of the meeting with enemy activity clearly audible. It would have been no wonder had the attendance been sparse but the meeting was extremely well attended, and the proceedings unhurried and unperturbed, surely the evidence of the gracious presence of the Lord. Two past students gave graphic pictures of medical work abroad. **Christine Cheal** spoke of her work in Nigeria where she had been able to hold clinics for leprosy sufferers and to manage a dispensary. In turn she had been able to give elementary instruction to national orderlies in medical practices and she said how wonderful it was to see them put this knowledge into action among their own people. **Frank Davies** told of the tremendous need of medical work in the villages of India and gave instances of how he had found the course at the MSM invaluable in his work amongst leprosy sufferers.

In his closing address, the Revd A. **Timothy Houghton**, himself a former student and prizewinner, spoke enthusiastically of the need for missionaries at that time, and in the future, to take advantage of the course which the MSM provided. He began by paying a personal tribute to the training he had received at the School, saying how valuable it had been in times of crisis in his own family, and how he had been able to deal with casualties at sea after being torpedoed en route to Burma.

He then went on to describe how his service, and that of colleagues trained at the MSM had been much enhanced by the knowledge gained there. Prior to the 2nd World War, Burma had a good system of government medical services, at least in the towns. There was a civil surgeon at the head of each district, and sub-assistant surgeons with their dispensaries in the smaller towns. However, in the more remote areas one soon found that efficient medical services only slightly touched the people, and missionaries like himself, were able to use the skills learnt at the MSM.

Mr Houghton again stressed the need for all missionaries to have similar skills because, not only were those skills needed in remote areas, but they could also be used in conjunction with professional medical work undertaken by doctors and nurses in the hospitals and medical centres (of Burma). At one time, when he had to take over the Mission administration in Upper Burma, he had to give up the medical work for which he was largely responsible. However, he found that he was still permitted to act as honorary anaesthetist in the hospitals and was able to help in many serious operations as a result of training received at the School. *'Whether one likes it or not'* continued Mr Houghton, *'it is essential for every missionary to undertake some form of medical work'.* One missionary who felt this to be relatively unimportant and who did not think it was necessary for her to go to the MSM had asked to be sent where there was an apparently efficient government medical service but when she returned to the UK for her furlough asked, as a priority, to be allowed to attend the MSM. On eventually returning to her station she found that as a result of her training she was able to gain entrance into many more homes than in her previous tour of service, so spreading more effectively the good news of the Great Physician, which is the aim of each student trained at the School.

Mr Houghton then went on to remind his audience of how our Lord went forth, and seeing the multitude was moved with compassion towards them, and healed many. Jesus could not see human sufferers without having the desire to meet their need. What a tragedy if we should go forth as missionaries, *'touching the ends of the earth'* and meeting an incredible amount of suffering, often due to ignorance, dirt and superstition, or heathen customs, or even as a result of war, and not be able to meet those needs. Those who have gone forth from the MSM have gone with greater confidence, knowing they will be the better equipped for definite action in helping to save life and relieving physical suffering, demonstrating the compassionate love of Christ, and so finding an entrance into many hearts with the gospel of Jesus which alone can save sinful men and women.

Speaking directly to the students about to leave, Mr Houghton said, 'I believe there is going to be an unprecedented opportunity for medical evangelism particularly in areas that have been devastated by war.' He spoke particularly of the countries of the Far East where there was an enormous amount of work to be done for the hundreds of unevangelized tribes, and where there had been a breakdown of medical services. He felt that particularly in Burma, the greatest opportunity for missionaries of all societies would be in the realm of medical evangelism.

In closing his address, Mr Houghton reminded his hearers of another occasion when our Lord was moved with compassion. *'He was moved with compassion when he saw the multitude distressed and scattered as sheep not having a shepherd'* (Matthew 9:36). He urged his listeners not only to increase their financial support for the School, but also to *pray* that the Lord of the Harvest would send forth labourers to meet the coming need and opportunity to 'preach and heal.'

Peace after Peril
During the next School session (1945-46) peace came to Europe during May, followed by peace with Japan *after the worst event the world has ever seen*, namely the dropping by the Allies in August of two atom bombs at Hiroshima and Nagasaki in Japan, with catastrophic effect.

Writing in the Annual Report for that year, the President of the School said:

> Now that the war is over, and the world open before us, there should be a great advance of all the Christian forces of this and other countries. The wounds of war are felt in all lands, and whilst much can be done in the way of giving material relief, the only real healing will come from the ministry of the gospel, accompanied by the healing of the body when inspired by the God of love.

Also during that year the Council was considerably strengthened by the addition of two new members, the Revd A.T.Houghton, the General Secretary of Bible Churchman's Missionary Society, and Mr Francis Stunt, a well-known solicitor. Almost a record number of students registered for the course numbering 41, of which 11 completed the full course. Some were missionaries on furlough, who had come to assess the value of medical knowledge in relation to their work overseas. Most had received previous training in theological or missionary colleges, and they were preparing to go to South America, China, India, Sudan, Kenya, Tanganyika and Ethiopia (after some repressive years of Italian occupation).

Again a very full curriculum was followed. The late Dr Edwin Neatby meant it to include everything that would be useful, and as the years progressed, constant watchfulness and revision were needed to ensure that it did not become overloaded. In 1945 this included Dentistry, the management and control of Tropical Diseases, Materia Medica covering both allopathic and homoeopathic medicines. General Pharmacy was taught, as was the dispensing of medicines. Every pioneer missionary had to prepare and dispense medicines at some time or other. Missionaries had also to be prepared for all kinds of emergencies and some instruction on how to make a diagnosis was of real value. First Aid to the injured and elementary Surgery were also prime essentials and these were taught with care and thoroughness and further instruction was provided by all the surgeons in the LHH. Dr Paul Brand, located at that time in central London, kindly stepped in to advise on the purchase of appropriate surgical instruments, as well as giving instruction in Anaesthetics.

The arrangement of students boarding at No.3 Powis Place in return for certain valuable services already noted, ceased on the termination of hostilities. So much kindness on numerous occasions was extended throughout this long period by Mr Knowles, the General Secretary of the LHH, as well as by the Board of Management.

The students had studied under many difficulties and at times under much strain and stress, but they seemed to think that a special urgency needed a special effort, and it was with real satisfaction that the General Council of the School reported in 1945 that the examination results had never been exceeded!

5 Post-War Recovery

The Year of the Cessation of War

1946 was the first year of peace after the long years of hostilities. It required many readjustments from everyone - indeed, the School's President referred to it by saying, 'It would be more correct to describe it as the year of the cessation of war'. War conditions had affected so many missionary areas of the world and yet, in spite of enormous difficulties, the witness to the gospel of our Lord Jesus Christ had continued. It was a matter of great thankfulness to Almighty God that the MSM was able to carry on its work with the minimum of disruption.

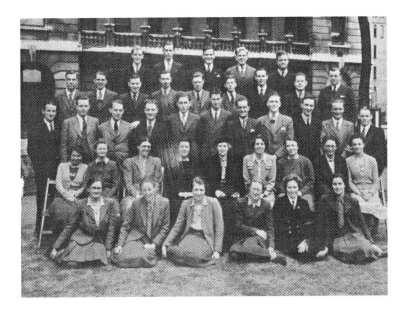

A Group of Students - June 1947

Back row: D.Nicholls, C.W.Callaway, G.Bell, P.P.Gammon, W.Gould,
Fourth row: D.Pape, W.Elliott, J.A.Kirk, A.Dexter, C.J.Ede,
R.R.Harter, W.Walker, A.Smyth, R.Duff,
Third row: N.J.Taylor, C.Moss, J.C.Cotterill, R.Hynds, P.Brandon, R.W.Lower,
A.J.Clarke, A.H.Gammon, W.W.Terrell, G.B.Cox, J.Black,
Second row: K.M.Ingle, A.L.Bates, M.Haines, Miss Harvey,
Miss Bargh, M.Stacey, M.Crooks, L.Webb, G.Dunkley,
Front row: A.S.McBurney, M.E.Thomas, P.Peters,
D.Robertson, A.Hocking, D.J.Griffiths,

With the cessation of hostilities, there came from all parts of the world a loud cry for re-inforcements. A great many young people in Great Britain responded and offered themselves to God's service. This meant a large intake of students at the School. In the five years through to 1950, nearly 200 took advantage of the medical training, many doing the full MSM course; *the largest intake of all being in 1947 when 48 were there!*

Pressure for Enlargement
This increase prompted the Council to approach the authorities of the London Homoeopathic Hospital for the renting of a larger room, which became available on the first floor of No.2 Powis Place, to serve as a lecture room. This was readily granted enabling the School to accommodate 12 extra students, though even so, with great reluctance, 20 more were turned away. However, the School's syllabus was such that lecture-room facilities were only part of the problem. Hospital work and experience meant the Council were careful not to take a larger number of students than the School could train adequately, as the emphasis was always on the practical application of the instruction given.

International Recognition of the MSM Certificate
Not all the students were from the UK. Most years, a few came from other countries, mainly from Sweden, South Africa, New Zealand and the USA, and it was gratifying to know that the training given was recognized by an increasing number of countries around the world. Writing from Nigeria in 1950, the Revd **Edward Bingham** said, 'You will be pleased to know that the certificate given me by the MSM has enabled me to get a medical permit and also an injection licence. These came through in record time, so we thank God for answered prayer and that the MSM's training is valued in high places.'

The Demobilization of Doctors
One great problem the School faced during the war years was the constant 'Call up' for military service of the doctors and other lecturers, particularly of the younger ones. Already in 1946, such personnel began to return and it was a cause for great cheer to know that nearly all of them were back again. Sadly a few had given their lives in the

cause of justice and human freedom and the School recognized their valour.

In the same year, the library was completely revised by Miss F.M. Caten, a trained teacher and librarian, who studied at the School throughout that session. As always, the Christian life of the School, and the fellowship with one another (and with others), was of a high order, and this was a great daily enrichment to everyone, the memory of it lasting for long years afterwards as a stimulating incentive, when serving on the various mission stations abroad.

Called Home

The School suffered the inevitable losses over this period as stalwart workers died. In 1948, the President for the previous 13 years, the Revd W.H.Aldis, passed to 'higher service'. Many warm tributes were paid to him and his loss was a great blow to the School. The report of his death in the Annual Report states simply: *'We shall miss him greatly - but while we mourn his loss we cannot but thank God for his friendship, his wise counsel and far-sighted leadership. He was indeed a true man of God.'*

During the same session, the School suffered another heavy blow through the death of Dr C.E.Wheeler, for many years a great friend and keen supporter of all its work. He normally presented the School Report for the Year at Annual Meetings and had been a member of the Council since 1934. He had also lectured at the School for very many years prior to that.

Yet another loss sustained during this same session was that of the Auditor, Mr T.Burton Miller: he too had been a good friend for many years.

A New President

Following the death of Mr Aldis in 1948, the Council invited the Revd A.T.Houghton MA, to become the President of the School - an invitation which was graciously accepted. The announcement of this appointment read as follows:

> Mr Houghton is a man of clear missionary vision; he has an intimate knowledge of the mission fields of the world, and considerable administrative and literary ability. He is a past student of the MSM having taken the course before going out to do pioneering missionary work in Upper Burma; thus he understands the outline of instruction we seek to give and its effectual working on the field. These qualities, and

a rich spiritual experience upon which he can draw, were factors which led the Council to conclude that Mr Houghton should be invited to follow the previous distinguished occupants of the office.

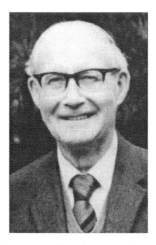

Canon A.Timothy Houghton
1896 - 1993

The Curriculum of the School

The following year (1949), the Council invited Dr J.C.MacKillop MB ChB, to become Clinical Tutor in place of the late Dr T.Miller Neatby. Shortly after his appointment, Dr MacKillop wrote a very helpful essay about the curriculum of the MSM which he sought to follow in his new work entitled, 'Achieving its Aim'. It went something like this:

> Briefly, the curriculum of the MSM aims to impart sufficient knowledge to enable the missionary to maintain health or to deal with illness whether in himself or in the national community in which he serves. In carrying out this aim it has to be remembered that, more often than not, qualified medical aid may be unobtainable and therefore the instruction should **not be too elementary**.
>
> In addition disease conditions met with may cover the whole wide field of medicine and so instruction given **must be comprehensive**.
>
> At the same time students themselves vary widely in educational background and natural aptitude, and so it is important that instruction **should be intelligible** to the slowest. Furthermore, the curriculum has to be compressed into nine short months, therefore instruction **must be intensive**.
>
> If we teachers have a measure of success in resolving these difficult conditions, it is the students themselves, who by their enthusiasm, make

it possible. Indeed, students often pass through an initial phase of mental indigestion or bewilderment, but this soon passes off, as soon as their interest is gained.

David Livingstone, one of the greatest missionaries who ever lived, was also a doctor and his medical knowledge proved an indispensible asset in carrying the light of Christian civilization through darkest Africa. Though this School makes no pretensions to turning out doctors in the ordinary sense of the word, the course is designed to inculcate confidence and self-reliance, based on knowledge, so as to enable students to deal satisfactorily with injury or disease when called upon to do so in the absence of qualified doctors.

The National Health Service

With the introduction of the National Health Service in 1947 the management of the MSM approached the immediate future with some trepidation. There was the possibility of all manner of limitations but under God's good hand, they did not materialize. The changes that did happen proved ultimately for the better, and the students continued to be received at the various hospitals as before.

A New Prize

Constant reference was made by those running the School to its co-founder and first Dean, Dr Edwin Neatby; his presence in leadership over so many of the early years made his name synonymous with the MSM. To perpetuate his memory a new prize was established in 1950 in honour of this great man: 'The Dr Edwin Neatby Prize'. The first recipient was Miss Irene King who later served with the Egypt General Mission and the prize consisted of a copy of *A Manual of Homoeo-Therapeutics* by Neatby and Stoneham, a case of surgical instruments and a hypodermic syringe.

More News from Overseas

Many letters from former students continued to be received by the Warden verifying the value of the courses the School offered. Miss **Mary Eccles** wrote from Tinnevelly in South India as follows:

You will be interested to learn that I am doing some medical work here, as well as language study, and I am happy to send you particulars of a few cases.

Patient No 1 had a skin disease for about 10 years and was unable to get it cleared up. One day she came crying to me about it. Her body was covered with sores the size of a pea or larger and full of pus. I hardly knew what it was but it did not take me long to decide to try

Sulphur, for she appeared to be a 'typical Sulphur patient'. I bathed the sores and applied some Sulphur ointment, but I also gave her a homoeopathic dose of Sulphur 200 and this treatment has produced a marvellous result. She is a different person now, neat and clean with a bright expression and the sores are almost gone.

Patient No 2 is a young lady of about 20 years of age with a threatened mastoid abscess: severe headache, high temperature, swelling and pain behind the ear, great discomfort and many symptoms vaguely expressed, which suggested to me Pulsatilla. A few doses were given of the 30th potency and shortly afterwards she was able to return to her work, for the inflamation resolved naturally.

Patient No 3 was a child of 4 years of age. He contracted pneumonia and was very ill and delirious with a very high temperature. The parents were most alarmed and sent to me for aid. Bryonia 30 was a great help and he recovered.

Patient No 4 was a mason working on the compound. He was lifting a heavy stone when it slipped and fell on his chest and injured him. He was in great pain and breathing in a distressed manner. I had no Arnica lotion but I painted the part with Iodine and gave him Arnica 6x. The pain gradually subsided and in a few days he came to see me, saying he was nearly well, and he brought his wife and another patient for 'medicine that cures quickly!' It is just grand to be able to help these people.

Royal Recognition

The London Homoeopathic Hospital celebrated its centenary in 1948. For many years the hospital had enjoyed royal recognition, having been granted a Royal Charter of Incorporation in 1928. In 1948 it had the honour of being granted permission to include the prefix *'Royal'* in its title, so becoming the Royal London Homoeopathic Hospital (RLHH).

A Most Dedicated Honorary Treasurer

The name of Sir John Weir appears in the earliest available literature of the Missionary School of Medicine going back to pre-World War I. He began as Chairman of the Medical Committee while a physician at the LHH and a lecturer on the Materia Medica. In the first report it was stated, 'Dr Weir is too well-known to require further mention and it is hoped that he will long continue his practical interest in the work and management of the School.' His service as Honorary Treasurer began in 1934 and continued for more than 30 years. Sir John was a popular lecturer in homoeopathy and being an obvious Scotsman was remembered each year at the AGM for his lengthy and original appeals for money.

The finances of the School were a constant cause for concern. 'Anxiety' is too strong a word but under the bountiful hand of God the needs were graciously met each year. In the days before World War II, a list of donors each year was printed in the Annual Report, but because of restrictions concerned with the conservation of paper during the war years, this practice had been dropped. In 1938, for instance, there were listed 121 donors, including subscribers, who together gave a little over £329. In 1932 there were 144 donors and subscribers giving £551. Most were quite modest amounts but each year there seem to have been one or two larger donations. In 1950, this figure rose to £813 with an extra sum of £500 being given as a legacy. Normally at each annual meeting, Sir John appeared to have painted a rather gloomy picture of the state of the School's financial position, due either to the fact that he was a careful and realistic treasurer, or simply because of his Scottish blood!

There is no doubt about it that throughout his long term of office, the MSM owed an enormous debt of gratitude to Sir John Weir for his loyal, enthusiastic and dedicated work for the School. He also attracted considerable support from the relatively well-to-do circle in which he moved.

In giving the Honorary Treasurer's report in 1948, Sir John revealed a slight increase in subscriptions and donations and expressed his thanks. He pointed out however, that these gifts by no means made up for the level of students' fees. 'But two kind friends came to the rescue!'

The Council had considered raising tuition fees but had voted against this in order to help prospective missionary applicants. The previous year, Sir John had suggested that every supporter of the MSM should also 'become an Honorary Treasurer'. Mr Francis Stunt, one of the Council members, gave an excellent example by taking up this challenge; so effectively that he himself collected the gratifying sum of nearly £300. This proved a great help on the year's working. 'But', said Sir John, 'efforts resulting in small amounts were also valued'.

Encouragements for the Students' Fellowship

By 1950 the Students' Fellowship was prospering and fulfilling a useful purpose. Through the Service Bureau a constant stream of medical necessities was flowing to the many different mission stations around the world. Life Membership - limited to past students and effected by the payment of two guineas - seemed to be increasing in popularity as each year many new members were welcomed into the Fellowship.

The Annual Report for that year stated: 'Past students will be interested to know that the MSM is planning a display at the Worldwide Evangelical Alliance missionary exhibition to be held in September in the Westminster Central Hall. Two students, David Chapman and Henry Mackay, have executed a splendid poster unsolicited, and to them we offer thanks. Photographs and other items will fill up the remaining space. Fellowship Day was grand: indeed these days are increasing in interest year by year and in spiritual depth and blessing. Greetings are sent from all at the School and prayerful remembrance from the Students' Fellowship Committee.'

World-famous Speakers

It must have become apparent by now that each session of the School concluded with an Annual Meeting normally held, until the 1960s, in the magnificent Examination Hall in Queen's Square (by kind permission). Reports of various kinds were presented, prizes awarded and talks given by ex-students on home leave. Ever since the School started many world-famous home and missionary visitors were being invited to this event to give a suitable closing message. Names such as, Bishop J. Taylor Smith, Mr A. Lindsay Glegg, Lord Radstock, Mr Montague Goodman, Mrs Howard Hooker, Bishop Frank Houghton, and Lady Dobbie appeared among those who had addressed the Annual Meeting.

These people are little known today but at the time were leading figures in the evangelical world. It should not pass unnoticed that the President of the School, the Revd A. Timothy Houghton was at that time the General Secretary of the Bible Churchman's Missionary Society (now known as Crosslinks) and also on the committee of the Keswick Convention (later serving as its Chairman for several years). There is no doubt that these links provided a ready access to many eminent missionary speakers, both men and women.

In 1932 and again in 1950, two famous intrepid spinster missionaries, **Mildred Cable** and Francesca French addressed the School at such meetings. For many years they had together trekked across vast areas in Tibet and the surrounding parts, preaching the gospel. At the 1950 annual meeting Miss Cable received a great welcome and prefaced her talk by saying that she was a convinced homoeopath, while waving a bottle of homoeopathic medicine aloft! She had seen many missionaries at work and had done medical work herself, and so understood how baffling situations could become. She stressed that often, through medical work, great victories for Christ had been won.

Miss Cable recalled an instance on the Tibetan border where a princess came to her house, riding along with her retinue which included a Tibetan Lama, and they all looked very downcast and melancholic. The princess's only son had been taken ill, and the prince had ordered them to take the child to the Christians for medicine and to obey all the instructions they were given. After examination, a diagnosis was made and the appropriate remedy given. In a few days the crisis passed and the child's life was saved. This opportunity gave access to a whole tribe for the preaching of the gospel.

Another instance occurred in a city in Central Asia where the missionaries, including herself, were badly received. Whips were flourished and they were pelted with stones resulting in bruising and injury. They knew the instigators were from the local mosque, and thus they were confined to their house by the behaviour of these men. One day, however, an elderly leader, with a long white beard and picturesque costume came to them. 'My wife is ill' he said, 'and I want you to come along and see her.' The request could not be granted because of the tense local situation. He at once took up the matter and it was agreed that the wife should receive the medical attention she needed. After she had recovered, the Chief was as good as his word and the missionaries - herself and Francesca French - were free to go where they would in the city without harm, and simply because *'With God's blessing, medicine had put the situation into a right relationship with the missionaries'*.

Miss Cable congratulated the students and wished them God's speed, reminding them that, as they looked to the Great Physician, they would find that he would work through their ministrations 'with signs following.'

Normal School Routine

Over the years the School's regular and normal routine became established practice, being followed to a greater or lesser degree each year. The Warden outlined this routine in 1951 as follows:

The course commenced in October and during that month basic subjects such as Anatomy, Physiology and Antisepsis were taught. We were pleased to welcome Mr Murphie FRCS to give these lectures and there was no fear that the students did not know their subjects well. As the course proceeded most elementary things medical and surgical were taught.

The surgical studies included First-Aid, General and Minor Surgery. Mr Tucker FRCS, Mr Cutner FRCS and Mr Dodd FRCS have together taken responsibility for this part of the curriculum and made a valuable contribution to the course. Mr Charles H. West of the St John Ambulance Association has demonstrated practical First-Aid and has been largely responsible for the high standard of efficiency the students have attained in this subject. Practical experience has been obtained in the Casualty Departments of several London hospitals, notably St Olave's Hospital in Rotherhithe, Poplar Hospital, Acton General Hospital and the RLHH. Thus the students are able to deal with accidents and emergencies with intelligence and confidence.

Dentistry is an important subject and Mr Hill has given his usual lucid lectures on this subject, which always appear to be very popular with the students. Clinical dental experience is gained in our own hospital (the RLHH) under the supervision of Mr Gillham, while Mr Clompus has most kindly consented to receive students at his dental clinics at Poplar and St Andrew's hospitals. The ability to provide relief from the pain of offending teeth, in areas where no dentists exist, is an incalculable asset to the missionary.

Elementary Medicine and Clinical Work is a comprehensive course. Case-taking and Diagnosis taught by Dr John MacKillop has been supplemented by his tutorials on the wards, when clinical features and important indications of disease are noted. Dr Percy Quinton and Dr Foubister give tuition in General Medicine and Children's Diseases respectively, and take great interest in teaching these subjects.

Homoeopathic Materia Medica is always taught alongside Medicine so that diagnosis and the necessary treatment are properly co-related. Dr Fairburn introduced students to the sources of drugs and the specimens of tree barks, seeds and leaves shown, always stimulated interest. Students have the option of attending the Honyman-Gillespie and Compton Burnett lectures given by Sir John Weir and others, a privilege they are not slow to seize.

A knowledge of elementary Dispensing is of great value and indeed essential when missionaries find themselves in circumstances where they must act on their own initiatives. General and Homoeopathic Dispensing has been given at the Royal London Homoeopathic Hospital. A special course for students hoping to serve in West Africa, and especially Nigeria, has been given by Mr Rawlings Elliot, the Chief Pharmacist at Charing Cross Hospital, to whom we are indebted.

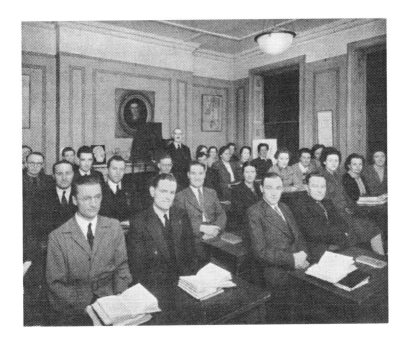

The Lecture Room During Tropical Diseases Course, 1947-48
The Lecturer, Dr. W.E.Cooke standing by the epidiascope

The Tropical section is in charge of two experts, Dr W.E.Cooke and Dr Charles Wilcocks; both have given their usual instructive lectures on Tropical Medicine and Tropical Hygiene respectively, and Dr Hartley has given excellent tutorials at the Seamen's Hospital at Greenwich. Again the students have attended the Wellcome Tropical Museum, which is quite near the School, and where first-class instruction material is laid out for students to observe, note and remember.

Certain special subjects are of importance and include Eye Diseases taught by Dr Pearson at the School, and by Dr Scoular at his clinic, and attendance at the Westminster Eye Hospital at Holborn, is permitted and is of immense value. Ear and Throat conditions are continually met with and Dr Cunningham has given tuition in both lectures and at his clinic. Mr Le Rossignol gives advice to students on Foot Health - very important to the students themselves. Dr Alva Benjamin gave superb instruction in Skin Diseases in his lectures and at his clinic at the RLHH. Miss Hall gave lectures on Obstetrics which were most helpful and permission was given to students - both *male* and female - to attend the General Lying-In Hospital at Waterloo by the Matron and her Board.

Lastly, we must extend our thanks to the Royal London Homoeopathic Hospital for the innumerable favours extended to us through the House Governor and Secretary, L.J.Knowles Esq, the Matron and her staff, also to the Regional Hospital Board. Sister Tutor and the Ward Sisters have been generous in teaching Nursing procedures and this has helped greatly as the examination tests show, revealing marked application on the part of the students, in fact all the doctors were especially pleased with the ability of the students and the high standard attained by them.

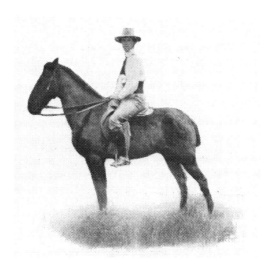

Revd A.S. McNairn

Recalling Long Service

On April 13th 1952 the death occurred of the Revd Stuart McNairn, the first registered student of the MSM way back in 1903. He was the General Secretary of the Evangelical Union of South America, and for some years served as a member of the Council of the School. Previously he had served as a missionary on that continent where he was able to use the medical knowledge which he had gained at the School.

After commenting on his passing, the MSM President went on to remind all its supporters that at the end of that year, the School would enter its Jubilee year. After giving a summary of how the School began, recorded in chapter 1, he made this interesting observation,

> It would appear that of the Officers, Council and Teaching Staff listed in 1911, only Sir John Weir, the present Honorary Treasurer, is still actively engaged in the work of the School which owes a great deal of gratitude to him for his genial help and inspiration throughout almost its whole history.

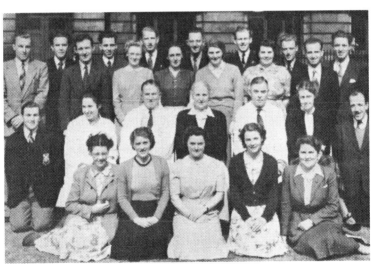

Some of the Students and Staff - 1951-52

Back row: I.J.Mckie, J.U.Davies, I.C.Timothy, D.Smith, A.Campbell, R.M.C.Beak,
M.Prior, H.Eisenhut, I.Campbell, E.Beresford, L.Gibbs, S.Wallace, H.Rosbottom,
Middle row: E.Orton, Dr.Marten, Dr.Templeton, MissBargh,
Dr.Kenyon, Miss Iveson, P.Downie,
Front row: F.Bedford, D.Stewart, E.Shakeshaft, M.Field, M.Fermand,

Another little point worth noticing was that Miss Evelyn Shakeshaft, who received the School Prize for that year, was a 'second generation MSM student' for her father, the Revd J.A.Shakeshaft took the MSM course when a young man.

Formalising School Precedents

A Constitution was drawn up and adopted by the Council in 1951 and printed for all to see. When successful students who completed the full course received their certificates they were required to sign the Declaration which read,

'I undertake not to practise in this country or to assume the position or title of a qualified Medical Practitioner at home or abroad.'

More Financial 'Headaches'

During that year financial anxieties were again a matter of concern. Sir John reported that during the year the Financial Committee had investigated the finances of the School and the honorary Auditor, Mr Metcalfe Collier, estimated a deficit on the year's working of £480. Mr Collier pointed out that the approximate annual cost of tuition for each student was £68, and the fee charged at that time was £25. This meant that the shortfall between actual cost and the fees paid by students inevitably resulted in a subsidy being taken out of public income. It was felt that the fees should be related to the actual cost of tuition and that they be raised to £63 for students able to pay the full amount. Those unable to pay this sum should be eligible for a 50% bursary.

The reader is reminded, that unlike today, few public grants were available to students studying for overseas missionary service. None was made by Local Education Authorities, although there were a few bodies which were helpful in this direction, especially certain Diocesan Missionary Associations.

Another financial problem concerned living accommodation in London for nine months of the year, which for many was likely to be an expensive matter, to say nothing of the daily bus and Underground fares to get to and from the School, as well as to the various hospitals around London for practical clinical experience. Then there were meals to be paid for, and laundry costs - public launderettes had yet to appear on the scene. However, these problems were just another part of *'learning to live by faith'* which is a normal feature of all missionary activity.

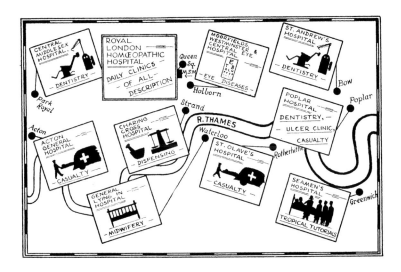

Chart Showing London Hospitals where Students
Gain Practical Experience

From the 50th annual report with the footnote,
Grateful acknowledgment to Philip Price, 'Clarke' prizeman 1953

Looking back over the years, all praise is offered to the Lord of the Harvest for his faithfulness and generous provision. Many students owed much to the Foreign Mission's Club in Aberdeen New Park (formerly in Clissold Park at Highbury). There, Miss Annie Angus, the warden for very many years (as was her mother before her!), wonderfully assisted by Miss Gladys Dawe, did a most gracious work, in not only running a 'hotel for missionaries on home leave, or in transit through the Capital', but giving accommodation to several MSM students at a most moderate rental. These students were made to feel wonderfully at home, even relaxing in the table-tennis room in the basement, and being kept well fed! These good ladies frequently turned a blind eye to hungry students in the dining hall going round for third-time helpings.

Encouraging Letters
Anyone tempted to question whether it was all worthwhile, has only to peruse some of the many letters - too many to include in this brief

history - which were received from ex-students working in far-flung outposts of the Christian Church around the world. Here are extracts from just a few.

The Revd **Kenneth Richardson** working with the Africa Inland Mission in Kenya wrote,

> With the nearest hospital 85 miles away..... we were living among a very needy people. Often we had brought to us those who had been mauled by leopards or gored by buffalo, many with severe tropical diseases such as malaria, dysentery, biharzia, yaws, hookworm and so on. Infants were also brought with all manner of illnesses and wasting diseases. Missionaries sent out to places like this without any medical knowledge - and in many parts of the world such places still exist today (1947) - is not only foolish but *criminal*.

Sister Schrader writing from the Solomon Islands in 1951 said,

> Here we have a Homoeopathic Mission Dispensary and during the last three years I have been alone, the nearest doctor being 300 miles away - it is not easy getting in touch with him.
> The medical knowledge and homoeopathic medicines have been a wonderful help and through the use of them I have been privileged to lead many people to Christ. All the national evangelists are trained in the use of homoeopathic medicines and they are wonderful in their prescribing; often their results are better than mine! When patients come to the dispensary it is often difficult to get the symptoms correctly as they speak in 'pidgin English' and a description of the pain may go like this, 'The pain go up leg belong me' or, 'Belly belong me sore' or, 'All down arm belong me'!
> Two years ago there was a big epidemic of whooping cough and over 1200 children died. In the area concerned every child under one year of age died, but in my particular district I only lost four, and one of those might not have died if the mother had been more careful. At present there is an epidemic of poliomyelitis and people are dying in great numbers. At our mission we are using homoeopathic drugs, especially Gelsemium, and people are improving.
> There was the little girl who had cerebral malaria. All the symptoms indicated the use of Bryonia, and I gave her a high potency. This initially resulted in a severe reaction but after an hour the child fell into a deep sleep and next morning the fever was allayed and the child gradually recovered. How I prayed and studied about this case. The father said, 'She get better you prayed used water medicine belong you.'

Mr **Dennis Nichol** wrote from Angola in Portuguese West Africa and told of a dramatic incident unconnected with homoeopathy. Remember, the MSM course covers some General Medicine.

One day the Angolan nurse came running up to the house. 'Sir, Tomasi wants you at the dispensary.' I ran along to find that he had fallen off his bicycle on to a tree stump, which had gone into his thigh making a gash as long as the forefinger and almost as deep. His friends had done their first-aid by putting unslaked lime all round the wound. You can imagine what happened with the moisture from the sore, as well as the pain Tomasi endured. Of course, cauterization had taken place even to the destruction of some of the flesh, for when he arrived it had all happened three days before!

I called up my colleague and we decided that we would suture it up. Needles were prepared but what were we going to use as an anaesthetic? We had some dental anaesthetic handy and so gave a local. The thigh was twice its normal size. However, after swabbing the outside with iodine we went ahead with stitching, leaving in the necessary drainage. The whole wound was then covered with sulphathiazole powder from three crushed tablets, and bandages applied. The next day when the patient was brought to us all swelling had disappeared. *'It was the Lord's doing and (to us) marvellous in our eyes.'*

1953: A Year of Celebration
'Fifty years of valuable and unique work!'
That was how the Council of the Missionary School of Medicine summarized the School's achievements at the commencement of the Fiftieth Session in 1953. It was hoped that entire year might be marked out in some special manner, particularly by increased interest and support on the part of the Christian public. Therefore, in that year, the Council set up a Jubilee Bursary Fund by which it was hoped to offer a number of entirely free places for students in financial difficulties and generous reductions in other needy cases.

It was further hoped that the great nationwide evangelistic enterprise, centred on London, with the visit of the American evangelist Dr Billy Graham, would result not only in the conversion of many to follow Christ in Britain, but also in awakening the church to a much greater zeal in world-wide missionary evangelism.

Another national event celebrated that year was the coronation of Her Majesty the Queen in Westminster Abbey. *Thus it was a season of celebration; and the MSM had so much to celebrate as well!* It rejoiced in God's provision in sending students from all nations of the world to study at the School, for it was not only inter-denominational but *international* and during those fifty years approximately 1300 students had received training; the majority of them having taken the full course.

Fifty years have now passed since the School celebrated the first fifty years. There is little doubt now that the years of Post-War Recovery were perhaps the hey-day of the School's existence. How blest it was at that time with its highest annual intake of students over several years and so many working together with immense sacrifice and dedication:

- lecturers and tutors who gave up their free time to help teach the students
- the ready availability of the RLHH in which the School functioned
- the successive matrons and all the staff under them
- the many hospitals and medical institutions in London always available
- the supporters, intercessors and donors, a host of gracious helpers
- and, perhaps most importantly of all, the succesive Council members and Officials of the School.

Sadly, in this Jubilee year, the loss was recorded of Dr Percy Quinton who died suddenly of a massive heart attack. He was for many years a member of the Council and for more than 20 years on the tutorial staff. He was a brilliant and natural lecturer with a warm personality that endeared him to the most nervous student. He was always ready to help the work of the MSM and was much beloved by each successive batch of students.

At the 1953 Annual Meeting in that Jubilee year, the School's Monitor, John Brown, speaking on behalf of the student body, voiced warm expression of thanks to the Doctors and Lecturers and said it had been an immense privilege to have sat at the feet of some of the country's leading physicians and specialists. He was confident that the students would always retain thoughts of gratitude to them, when, God willing, on their mission stations overseas in future days they were dealing with sick and needy people.

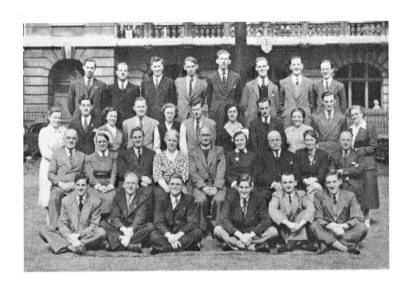

Some Officials and Coronation Year Students - June 1953

Back row: J.A.Brown, H.F.Fox, A.Fraser, J.R.Rutland, P.Price, E.C.West,
W.McKeown, C.Bruins,
Third row: A.L.Antturi, D.S.Lock, S.G.Jones, K.J.Jansen, D.M.Husband,
D.A.Husband,
E.M.Flory, W.S.Todd, K.R.Ashcroft, L.H.Dent, E.H.Raisenan,
Second row: Dr.W.E.Cooke, Sister Lyle Bottom, F.F.Stunt,
Miss Bargh (Warden & Secretary), Rev.A.T.Houghton (President),
Miss MacKenzie (Matron RLHH), Sir John Weir (Honorary Treasurer), Miss Iveson,
Dr.J.C.MacKillop,
Front row: K.Ashcroft, J.R.Harbinson, E.H.Wilks, L.C.Powell, D.A.Herm,
L.C.H.Clifton,

A Disappointing Decade

Having completed in 1953 the fiftieth Jubilee year of the founding of the School, the future was looked forward to with renewed expectation. The President referred to the possibility of an increase in missionary candidates as a result of the Greater London Crusade led by Dr Billy Graham from America which had just concluded. However, during 1955 the School was only half full of students, which apart from anything else, meant that financially MSM was far from being viable. This shortage of students was to become a matter of increasing disappointment as the decade wore on. Nevertheless, in spite of this problem, the School carried on as usual. No fewer than 24 tutors gave expert tuition in the Lecture Room with many other professional staff helping with practical assistance in the clinics as well.

Notable Retirements

Sadly, during the 1955 session, the School relunctantly said goodbye to Dr Thomas Pearson who lectured on Eye Diseases for over thirty years. His was a subject very important to missionaries, as we have seen, and hundreds of former students remember him with gratitude. Also during that year, Dr Charles Wilcocks at the Bureau of Tropical Hygiene felt obliged to relinquish his lectures due to an overfull programme. He gave lucid instruction on Tropical Hygiene. His splendid book *Health and Disease in the Tropics* remained a continuing source of help long afterwards. The author of this history will long be thankful for the doctor's advice. Some years later, when on safari in a remote area of N.W.Kenya, he awoke one morning and was about to put on his boots, when he recalled Dr Wilcocks saying, 'When in the tropics, always shake out your boots before putting them on.' He did this, and out dropped a large scorpion!!

A Royal Bouquet

The RLHH was honoured by a visit of HM The Queen on November 10th 1955. The occasion was in celebration of the bi-centenary of the birth of Dr Samuel Christian Hahnemann, the founder of the Homoeopathic system of medicine. Before beginning her tour of the Hospital Her Majesty was presented with a bouquet of flowers, leaves and berries arranged in the form of a handbag, with a cord handle for carrying. Included in the bouquet were 54 specimens of plants used in the preparation of medicines and particularly homoeopathic medicines. They were all collected from the home of Dr Margery Blackie at Hedingham Castle. She was later to succeed Sir John Weir as a Homoeopathic Physician to the Queen. Dr Helena Banks prepared the bouquet which was photographed to form the cover of Dr. Margery Blackie's book - *The Patient not the Cure*, (now out of print).

It was regrettable that Sir John Weir, the School's Honorary Treasurer and the Senior Consultant to the Hospital, was unable to be officially present owing to an accident. However, the Queen paid her Physician a visit in his private room at the Hospital.

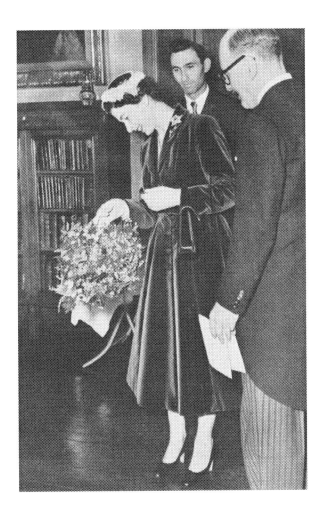

Her Majesty the Queen admiring the bouquet presented to her
on the occasion of her visit to the Royal London Homoeopathic Hospital,
November 10th 1955

The Boake Trust

Throughout its life the MSM owed an enormous debt of gratitude to many friends and supporters, some titled, many not, some highly skilled and professionally well qualified, others 'just ordinary folk' who gave without stint of their time, their prayers, their expertise and their money. On November 20th 1956 there was laid to rest one of the greatest benefactors of the School, Mrs J.G.Boake, who for many years served as a member of the Council. Both in her lifetime and beyond there was generous support to students through The Boake Trust, the assets of which now form part of the Endowment Fund.

Although from her own nursing experience Mrs Boake could appreciate the value the course provided, her interest was maintained and enhanced because she had a right sense of spiritual values. It was never the intention of the School to send overseas men and women equipped solely to relieve physical suffering, but to use the knowledge acquired to show the love of Christ for all in need, whether physical or spiritual. In the words of a hymn sung at Mrs Boake's funeral, past students all over the world are able to proclaim, 'Jesus, the sinner's Friend' in the most effective way by showing their own sympathy with, and desire, and ability to meet human need.

Grateful as the Council was for the help given by such benefactors as Mrs Boake, yet as Sir John Weir often pointed out, the financial stability of the School would have been better assured by the regular giving of smaller amounts by a larger number, than by the substantial gifts of a few generous-hearted friends.

An Experiment
A new idea was tried by the School in 1956 that later proved to be of considerable advantage to its future development. This was '*A SHORT COURSE*' for missionary candidates who were able to attend a brief series of lectures only, rather than doing the whole nine-month course.

Former Student Honoured
In that year, the Council received a newspaper from Nassau informing them of the award of the MBE insignia being given in the Queen's Birthday Honour List, to an ex-student of the MSM, **Walter Kendrick**, at a private investiture at Government House, by His Excellency the Governor, the Earl of Ranfurly, for *'Valuable and most unselfish service during more than fifty years'*. Mr Kendrick was the first person ever to be licensed by the Governor as an *'unqualified'* medical practitioner in the Outer Islands.

Importance of a Correct Diagnosis
Much sacrificial service was constantly being given to the School on the part of the doctors and other lecturers. At this time, for instance, Dr

John C. MacKillop set aside one complete afternoon a week for six months of the nine month session to give students clinical instruction in diagnosis and elementary medicine, on the wards.

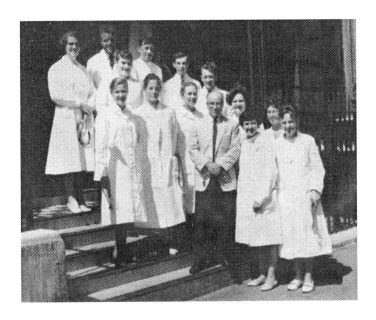

Ready for 'the Round'!
Dr. MacKillop's Tutorial Class, 1962-63

Back row: Y.R.Stofberg, M.I.Hunter, W.Loffelhardt,
Third row: D.Tonge, J.D.Crisp, C.L.Rawlins,
Second Row: S.Peltola, R.Moser, E.H.Hokkanen, D.Shaw,
Front row: Dr. MacKillop, P.O.Sills, D.M.Oakey, H.Blessing,

Mr **Gottfried Schalm** of the Sudan Interior Mission wrote from Northern Nigeria to the Secretary of the MSM in 1957 about the importance of this aspect of the training.

> Only recently, a man came to me and he had a pain in his abdomen. He had had no stools for five days. He wanted me to give him an aperient, but I hesitated for I thought of intestinal obstruction. When I saw him again in the evening I decided the diagnosis was an obstructed and strangulated hernia. I got him on my motorcycle and took him to the nearest hospital at once, and he was operated on the same night. Now he is back again and very well. *To make a correct diagnosis is often a matter of life and death to a patient.*

6 A Monitor's Memories

'"Blankets....Tuppence each!!"' So the newspaper vendors shouted in a desperate attempt to sell off their remaining papers.

It was around midnight on a cold wet evening in early June 1953 along the road bordering London's Hyde Park. The whole area was agog with excitement as hundreds of people of all ages occupied every available space in order to watch the many processions due to pass along that road the following day when HM Queen Elizabeth II attended her Coronation in Westminster Abbey. All who were able, lay down full-length on the hard wet pavement, in order to try to get some sleep. This was well-nigh impossible, except perhaps, for those who were stone deaf!

Then, suddenly the atmosphere changed dramatically as the enterprising newspaper vendors took advantage of a further news development:
'Everest conquered!....Read all about it!' they shouted.

Everybody stirred, and soon there were queues forming to buy a paper. It was the first time in history that anyone had climbed the highest mountain in the world and survived to tell the world. Everyone was eager, even at that late desperate hour, to get first-hand information about it.

One such group along that Hyde Park road that particular night was a number of students who had just completed the fiftieth session of medical study at the MSM before dispersing to all parts of the world. The Coronation was an event which permitted them to enjoy one last day together. The Queen's crowning was celebrated by millions around the world, but to those involved, the completion of the 50th session at the MSM was cause for high praise to our great Lord and King, Jesus Christ.

The author of this history was one of those students. Nearly 50 years later he contacted the Monitor of that session, John Brown, to try to recall some of his memories of that year of study and training. John kindly agreed and this is what he wrote:

How we lived
There must have been a wide variety of experiences amongst us students, such as financial stringency, long distance travelling, good and bad lodgings. However, I do not recall many details, apart from

personal ones and those of my room-mate, Ernie Wilks. During the first term-and-a-half he and I lodged at Walthamstow, a distance of five miles from the School. The daily journey by cycle was daunting in spite of the blessings of youthful fitness and enthusiasm. The early start for 9 o'clock lectures still prompts a vague recollection of chill and numbness.

The route, carefully worked out on an ancient 'London A to Z' included Essex Road, Upper Street Hackney, past the old Sadler's Wells Opera House, a side route through Lamb's Conduit, and finally to Great Ormond Street and Powis Place. In those early 50s the London trams had gone but not all the tramlines. We learned to steer our bikes across them at a wide angle to avoid disaster! One student, David Lock, had equipped his cycle with a quaint, post-war power pack which had a roller operating directly on to the rear tyre.

A small contingent of students lodged comfortably, congenially and cheaply at the Foreign Missions' Club then situated at No.5 Clissold Park in Highbury (since demolished). In the second term, Ernie Wilks and I joined them. I vividly recall the sense of profound thankfulness for the atmosphere and facilities of that long-established Christian institution where, besides various categories of Christian students and serving missionaries, lodging for a night or two whilst in transit across London, a few gracious elderly missionaries lived in retirement. Young and old, we were a happy, supportive community. Miss Angus, the manager, who had apparently always lived there, recalled riding her tricycle in and out of the dining rooms as a little girl. One of the duties of her deputy, Miss Dawes, was to arrange the guests' individual napkin rings. This was done in such a way as to ensure that the community 'mixed around' and did not get into cliques. Nevertheless she was adept at setting the married and the one or two single ones together. It used to be a matter of some levity that Miss Dawes had people's romantic destiny in her hand with those napkin rings!

For some, the journey 'home' was regularly by Underground from nearby Russell Square. I have an impression of Harold Fox and Philip Price walking along Queen's Square in that direction - Philip's umbrella immaculately rolled as it always was.

Apart from lectures, clinics and study, the heart of student life was lunch in the Library. The scene was always one of lunch papers, coffee mugs and continuous conversation. I do not recall any disputes, rows or factions; there always seemed to be an accepted high standard of Christian fellowship.

For me, that year at MSM was my first experience of living in London and this in itself was a landmark experience. It was life in a new dimension: the daily presence of busy London streets, buildings and traffic, the frequent charging off in all directions by cycle - often considerable distances - to clinics at far-distant hospitals. My most memorable recollection is of the night when Ernie Wilkes and myself arranged to sleep at the School in order to be on hand to go over to the Lying-In Hospital where a birth was imminent. The strategy worked and we were present to witness our first birth.

The student body, six women and nineteen men, which included two married couples, was far from being a staid and solemn lot. Pranks and escapades happened; spirits ran high one day in the lecture room when no staff were present and study seemed far from the thoughts of the majority. Jeremy Rutland climbed out of the first floor lecture room window and down the drainpipe into the street below. Laurie Clifton found some excuse to fetch a bowl of water and tip it out of the open window - one hopes, not on top of Jeremy!

What Lectures were Like

My recollections are decidedly positive. This, I believe, is largely due to the personality and standard of the lecturers. Many of them were giants in their field and it was a once-in-a-lifetime privilege to hear and be with them. The lecture material was fascinating: medicine, for many of us was a new world to explore. We were quite a large study group that year and the lecture room at No.2 Powis Place was quite full. Lecture attendance must have been good. The room was equipped with a skeleton, always carefully draped when not being studied - it was given a name which I have forgotten. Laughter, quips and repartee were a feature with some lecturers. There were idiosyncracies among them. Dr Kenyon, lecturer in Homoeopathic Materia Medica, who always attended with his secretary, invariably insisted upon all the windows being open. He used to take the opportunity to remark that this was a characteristic of Carbo Vegetabilis. There was frequently a great rush to open all the windows before he blustered into the room. Dr Kenyon often declared his intention of devoting his declining years to the compilation of a Comparative Homoeopathic Materia Medica. I wonder if it was ever written.

Lectures in the Boardroom of the RLHH were another thing altogether. They were shared with the medical post-graduate students who were reading for their FFHom. Here, Sir John Weir was undoubtedly one of the unforgettable figures. He had a light, dainty step as he entered, always immaculate in black jacket and pin-stripes, as if he had just returned from the Palace and attending the Queen, as, of course, he did on occasions. Sir John had his favourite stories, one of which was about the 'Blimey Bed' in the Homoeopathic Hospital. It had originated when Queen Mary visited and was involved in some basic conversation with an East End patient.

An American lady doctor frequently attended Sir John Weir's lectures and was known for her forwardness at question time with a familiar, 'But, Sair John?'

A favourite story told by Dr Twentyman was 'The Brown Paper Remedy,' a Case Study of a very successful treatment of a lady patient. It included her reference to some homely remedies which she had tried. Her own conclusion about her cure was that, 'It must have been the brown paper in which they were wrapped'!

How We Coped with Clinics

Clinics were perhaps, the most meaningful point of encounter on the Course. How could it be otherwise? We were young, inexperienced lay-people (at least as far as medicine was concerned). We were at the beginning of a brief medical training, of which as we all know, many past graduates of the School, by the grace of God, made outstanding use. But we were novices being brought face to face with patients, many of whom were in an hour of crisis. What must they have thought and felt, and what did we!? A few instances of impatience and annoyance and even crisis are recalled, as when a student mentioned the name of a disease which we had been forbidden to mention during a ward round. On one occasion a doctor excluded the attending students from a clinic until they had learned more physiology!

The many values of these clinics, however, included a new awareness of people in various conditions of pain and distress; the skill and professionalism of doctors and surgeons in administering the healing art - including homoeopathy - and the effects, sometimes before our eyes as, over a period, we saw patients returning to clinics, relieved and cured.

Students were sometimes involved in quite surprising medical situations like extracting teeth, giving intra-muscular injections, testing urine, (trying) to take blood pressure, and treating wounds and minor accidents, with staff at hand to refer to, of course, in several hospital casualty departments. Would all this have been possible today? Were we fortunate? I think we were!

Dr Muriel Adams, one of the Clinicians, was a devout Christian who devoted some of what leisure she had to running a Sunday School. She clearly welcomed students and was well aware of the evangelistic work to which they were heading. During spare minutes in the clinic (were there any of these?) she would seek to enhance our lecture-room knowledge. 'What shall we talk about', she would say, 'will it be the circulation of the blood?'

Study

Clearly some enjoyed and coped with study better than others. There were very different attitudes to it. Some felt it a Christian duty to give the utmost attention to it. Jeremy Rutland said he spent most of his time reading the Bible and, to be sure, his Bible was open on his desk most of the time. I do not recall that he had any particular problem in keeping up with what he was supposed to know. Others seemed to feel that, come what may, evangelistic activities must always come first.

Before exams a small coterie of students would burn the midnight oil - and the small hours - in the comfortable library at the Foreign Missions' Club. One in particular said his object was to draw off a summary of all his lecture notes and then to endeavour to learn that. In spite of all these efforts, and perhaps some others which were not so strenuous, results must often have fallen below what some lecturers and examiners required. In reply to the Monitor's letter of thanks for his services, Dr Twentyman said that he 'enjoyed teaching the students, although at times it seemed that a hammer might be necessary' and when berating the student body for comparatively poor examination results, he expressed amazement that 'no one, not even one, had remembered the cold sweat of Veratrum Album'. Of course, we have all remembered it ever since! After all, we were, in a sense, competing with fully trained doctors.

Christian Activities

The religious, evangelical and evangelistic emphasis has been strong and clear in the policy of MSM from the beginning. In our year, 1952-53, a period was set aside every week for a Students' Prayer Meeting and there were also regular meetings to which a missionary or Christian leader came to speak with a view to deepening our devotion and extending our vision.

Active evangelism was also part of the programme with a regular Open Air Meeting at a site in Clerkenwell (if I remember correctly). Paramount in this activity were Kenneth and Kathleen Ashcroft who felt a particular call to evangelism in the personal and open air spheres. Kenneth once told us how, in his experience in London prior to attending the MSM, he got deeply involved one day talking to an individual in the precincts of the Royal Courts of Justice in the Strand. The conversation got loud enough to disturb a Court in session and the Judge sent a message to Kenneth and his contact! 'Move on.' Ken did not seem to regard this as being anything extraordinary.

Individual students were occasionally engaged in preaching or other Christian work of their choice and interest. Ted West encouraged involvement in a weekly evangelistic meeting in Deptford. It was his practice to call out as students were preparing to leave at the end of the week: 'Friday night, Fellowship bright!'

Christian activities included student input to the annual Fellowship Day which was a regular event for many years (to do with the Students' Fellowship). In our year, David Lock, who was an accomplished choirmaster - he must have been exceptional to weld together both musicians and non-musicians (I was one of the latter) - formed and trained a male voice choir to sing at this event. The piece, as I so well remember, was 'Sweet is the work my God, my King' to the tune 'Deep Harmony'. It was the only time I ever sang in a choir.

Sunday evening Ward Services at the RLHH were held regularly during term time. The only incident which I recall is, unfortunately, a negative one. In a prayer, mention was made of a gravely ill patient and the Ward Sister was incensed and forbad further services on her ward. Following these services the students would sometimes attend the Nurses' Christian Fellowship meetings held in the basement of the Nurses' Home on the opposite side of Great Ormond Street. The speaker at one of these was H.K.Hine, who translated from Russian the well-known hymn 'How great Thou art' and whose daughter Sonia would later enrol for training at MSM. I recall him playing it most enthusiastically on the piano.

Social Activities

Rather surprisingly perhaps, amongst the students' officers appointed at the beginning of the School year were two Social Secretaries. The outings they arranged were only occasional. The only one, apart from the end of year outing, which I can remember, was to the Tower of London. The last outing of our session had a particularly relaxed and celebratory atmosphere. It was a boat trip on the Thames. The impression lodged most firmly in my mind about this event is of one of our most diligent students, Alistair Fraser, reading to us all, extracts from 'Winnie the Pooh'. He knew how to study but also how to relax!

The author is much indebted to John Brown, Monitor of the 50th session, for writing his memories of 'day by day' practicalities. John was a fine Monitor, always helpful, conscientious and bearing a fine Christian testimony.

In **How We Coped with Clinics** *John Brown refers to a doctor whose personal story is a fine illustration of the value and influence of a life fully surrendered to God. The following testimonial has been provided by Miss Ann Whitaker M.A.(Oxon.), to whom the author is also indebted.*

Dr Queenie Muriel Frances Adams, MRCS, LRCP, MFHom. (1902-1999)

Dr Adams always knew she was meant to be a doctor. But in those days girls stayed at home and it was still fairly exceptional for a woman to have a career. Coming to the Lord as she did at a CSSM beach mission in 1920, when she was 18, God immediately called her to speak to others of her Saviour, and after some difficulty, in 1928 she was at last able to go to Redcliffe Missionary Training College, then at Chiswick. Called to go out to Egypt in 1931, she worked first with the Church' Mission to the Jews, and later with the Egypt General Mission, as a teacher.

A fellow missionary developed a bad abscess which did not respond to orthodox treatment. Dr Adams used to say, 'I remembered that my mother used to be interested in homoeopathy and had taken us to homoeopathic doctors when we were ill. A friend of mine in the Egypt General Mission was running a homoeopathic clinic not far away and with her treatment, my colleague's abscess soon healed. I began to take Jewish people who were enquiring into Christianity to the clinic when they had something the matter with them. Again and again treatments were successful. "If I am ever in England long enough," I said to myself, "I'll try to take the same medical missionary course that she took".'

Invalided home, she enrolled at the Missionary School of Medicine. This was a turning point in her life. It was then that doctors said to her: 'You should take a full course and become a doctor, shouldn't you?' Her response was, 'I know.' She often spoke in later years of her appreciation of that one year course at the MSM.

But how to come by the full training in medicine? There were no grants for medical students at that time. Dr Adams had not taken money from her parents for many years, nor had she had a formal education, or taken any public examination. However, she applied to the Royal Free Hospital and was accepted. She was 35 years old. The condition was that she must gain her matriculation (equivalent to A-levels) in the first year.

God wonderfully provided for her general finances and for a splendid microscope. But on that first day as a student, she walked into the Royal Free with only a penny in her pocket. 'I think I shall just write a cheque for these textbooks we have to buy', said a well-to-do student. 'I don`t think I`ll do that', said Dr Adams. But the Lord provided. Half way through her training, there was opportunity to apply for a scholarship. She had not quite realized that there would be so many details about herself to be entered on the application form, but, as she often said later, the column on 'sources of income' was the easiest sum she had ever had to do. 'Nil' was the total. At the bottom of the form she wrote, 'My God shall supply all your need according to his riches in glory by Christ Jesus' (Philippians 4:19). This caused a sensation when she was later interviewed by the committee. 'How have you managed?' they asked. She was able to speak to them of God's wonderful way of providing. They then gave her two scholarships!

She often spoke of the kindness to her of all her teachers. Of course, she was longing to help people medically and started to treat, homoeopathically, one or two people she knew. She charged one shilling for a consultation. In a short space of time she was running a clinic in North London, in the sitting room of a minister and his wife. This was not, of course, in order and as the clinic grew she became embarrassed at the thought that discovery might lead to criticism of the Royal Free Hospital, which had been so good to her. She had to call a halt to the work.

Then came the war and after it a determination not to work within the Health Service, but to trust the Lord for a private practice. When she qualified, Mrs Douglas Porter, widow of a former secretary of the Egypt General Mission, gave Dr Adams a copy of Kent's (homoeopathic) Materia Medica, which had belonged to Dr G.H.Baring Deck, a well-known missionary doctor who had run a missionary hospital ship in the South Sea Islands. Mrs Porter wrote in the front of the book for Dr Adams: 'May medicine be the true handmaid of the Gospel.' This had always been Dr Adam's prayer.

As the years went by, the practice flourished, as she held clinics not only in her rooms in Harley Street, but in Reading (visited weekly), in Hastings, Wimborne and Bournemouth (each visited monthly) and Jersey (from time to time). Her modest fees were reduced when people could not afford them. Her joyful activity and energy were enormous and only eternity will reveal the number of souls who came to Christ through her ministry. Sometimes she prayed for years for patients before the Lord showed it was the right time to speak to them sensitively of spiritual things. She loved work with children. A special interest was the autonomic nervous system, and when invited to speak at a meeting of 'Caring Professions Concern' in North Wales some years ago she chose, instead of giving a spiritual message, to read a paper she had written describing the function and dysfunction of the Autonomic Nervous System, which she regarded as meriting much more attention than was usually paid to it by the medical profession.

Moving to Cornwall in 1965, medical and spiritual work continued from her home at Tremore Manor, near Bodmin. As a student at the MSM she had appreciated the opportunity to learn from Dr Margaret Tyler at the Royal London Homoeopathic Hospital about manipulation and there were dramatic moments during her clinics. A St John's Ambulance brought a patient one day, a car mechanic who had injured his back at work some time previously and was not making progress. He was in agonies of pain and had been given 'gas and air' during the journey. Dr Adams went into the ambulance and, after examination, manipulated the patient, who was then able to climb the staircase to her consulting room. He was back at work two weeks later. His aunt, chronically suffering, then came along. Patients were always recommending their friends to consult her, sure that they would be helped. 'Brilliant, unconventional and limitlessly kind', was the description of her by one doctor.

In recent years she was grieved by the ignorant criticism of classical homoeopathy as associated automatically with the occult. She wrote a paper vigorously opposing this view, distressed that a system of medicine used by missionaries world-wide for so many years to assist their families and those they were seeking to win for Jesus, should be ostracized in this way. 'But it has always been like that with homoeopathy - people have always tried to oppose it', she would say, peaceably, and continued unswervingly to put her full confidence in it, as she had from the time of her course at the MSM. Patients stayed with homoeopathy too, sometimes families of three generations.

Her patients were all over the world and many continued to consult her almost to the end of her life. One, writing shortly after her death, said 'She must have been 95 years old when she cured my knee!'

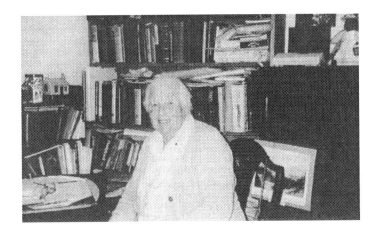

Dr. Queenie M.F. Adams
1902 - 1999

7 Student Enthusiasm

Inside No 2 Powis Place

No 2 Powis Place, home for the MSM during the years of the School's life was normally a hive of activity for both staff and students, and agility, both physical and mental was essential. The old Georgian house frequently shook with the bounding bouyancy of youth!

Those stairs!

There were three long flights of them soaring steeply, each above the other to reach the various floors, with cloakrooms and other departments going off from each landing. Students in their prime bounded up them two at a time, whilst more senior lecturers and council members, and others, paused, puffing considerably, once the third flight was conquered. The author is old enough to remember both experiences!

The students of Session 55 (1957-58), had so much surplus energy, that in addition to leaping up and down the stairs with great heartiness every day, they showed something of their appreciation to the staff, doctors and nurses who lectured them by decorating the Lecture Room. Not only did they execute the work with efficiency, they also defrayed the cost of the materials, much to the delight of their much-loved Honorary Treasurer and lecturer, Sir John Weir. The redecoration 'was certainly needed' and soon made the whole room look 'so neat and efficient'.

And to end the year, this extra-energetic student body had a rousing Christmas party.

'The Library had been given a festive air; candles twinkled amidst holly and evergreen; the table was laden with good things, and on it reposed a delicious looking cake decorated with coloured icing and bearing the arresting insignia "*Similia similibus curentur*". (Appropriate for the occasion but not to be administered in the "infinitesimal" dose!) Guitarist and songsters rendered "*An Ode to the MSM*" which was clever and amusing. Later games were played and carols sung. It was an evening of happy entertainment interwoven with the inspiration of the immortal story of the birth of the Saviour.'

Another Special Cake

After the Council meeting in early November 1958, a tea had been arranged, with a birthday cake as the central attraction. A few friends were also permitted to attend, together with the staff and students. It was to mark the 80th birthday of Sir John. When justice had been done to the excellent repast, the President reminded all present of the warm and sustained interest Sir John had shown in the work of the School almost from its beginning, having served as a member of the Council for 41 years, much of that time as the Honorary Treasurer. Sir John was asked to accept a silver salver suitably inscribed to mark the occasion. In responding, Sir John thanked everyone for the delightful surprise given to him that afternoon and said he was glad to have been associated with such a far-reaching and splendid work as the Missionary School of Medicine.

Perhaps not to be outdone by their immediate predecessors, the students of the next session (1958-59) supplied and fixed a new double-ringed gas stove in the students' kitchen and the Monitor himself (George Martin) chose to stay on after the completion of the course to redecorate both the students' and the staff's kitchens, so that they 'looked quite resplendent in their new coats of paint'. This thoughtfulness and achievement was noted by the Council and Staff with warm acceptance and thanks.

Nigerian 'Check-Out'

As usual, the students for this session came from many countries including America, Australia, South Africa, Germany, Holland and Switzerland. Most of them had already received theological and missionary training in their respective countries before joining the MSM. Two of them were on furlough - they were two hospital sisters from Nigeria.

Previous to the session, the School received a special overseas visitor. He was Dr. Rowson, who was Head of the Pharmacy Department of the Nigerian College of Arts, Science and Technology in Ibadan. He was deputed to report to the Pharmacy Board in that country on the arrangements at the MSM. Fortunately, he seemed well satisfied with all that he saw.

Future Council Members

By a strange coincidence, two former students of the MSM spoke at the Annual Meeting in 1959. Thirty-five years later both were serving the MSM as Council members. They were Mr Alfred Lodge who served as President, and the author of this history.

Alfred Lodge served with the Brethren Assemblies Mission at Idah in Northern Nigeria. In the autumn of 1939 he arrived at Queen's Square (adjacent to the MSM) on a bicycle, having cycled from his home in Yorkshire! Whilst on this rather epic journey he stopped at Oxford, where a telegram caught up with him stating that an anonymous donor had given £500 to the School in a bid to keep it open. Owing to the outbreak of World War II there was uncertainty as to whether or not the School would be able to continue to function. The Council not only took this generous gift as a sign that the School should carry on, but awarded this entire amount to Alfred as a bursary to pay for the cost of his training!

In those dark and difficult days it was impossible to see what would happen but the course began and nine months later, it concluded. Soon Alfred found himself on a boat in a convoy of ships bound for Nigeria and was wondrously preserved on a dangerous voyage. On arrival at the mission station he found a large medical work in progress, for the medical needs of the people were immense and no fewer than 10,000 were being treated every year.

Alfred spoke at the 1959 meeting of one patient he particularly remembered from those early days of his service.

> A little lad named Bako was brought many miles through the forest to the mission by his sister and over his head I noticed a filthy cloth. When I removed it I found, as I had guessed, his poor little eyes streaming with pus, a most pathetic sight. I began to bathe and irrigate his eyes regularly day by day and to apply suitable antiseptic cream, and after many weeks we had the joy of seeing his eyes healed and he was able to see once more. But a greater joy was in store for us, for Bako, who had heard repeatedly each day of the Lord Jesus Christ, wanted Him for his Saviour also, and as we knelt and prayed together, so simply, little Bako passed from spiritual death unto eternal life.

The author of this book, having served with the Bible Churchman's Missionary Society (now known as Crosslinks), also spoke at that meeting, recounting his early experiences among the Pokot people of North West Kenya. I subsequently wrote a book entitled *God in the Valley,* from which the following extract is taken:

> Sometimes the safaris I made were for medical reasons. Before I came to Kenya I had spent a year at the Missionary School of Medicine in London learning some of the rudiments of dispensary work, and this gave me some good opportunities to reach the people with the gospel through medical help. One morning a boy called Lokong, son of the local headman, arrived at my tent. He greeted me in the normal way.
>
> 'Can you help me?' he asked.

'What is it you want?' I replied.

He fidgeted uneasily on one leg, resting the other on its kneecap in the usual Pokot fashion and balancing his body on his staff.

'Yesterday, my father had drunk much komun (honey beer) and was staggering about like a camel', he explained. 'At the home-coming of the cows he went to his farm to cut down a tree so that the millet would grow tall. He was slow in getting himself clear as the tree fell and a branch pinned him to the ground, making a deep gash in his leg'.

'Where is he now?' I asked.

'Sitting grumbling at the door of his hut. He sent me to call you as he cannot walk', Lokong replied.

The headman's house was about three miles away and I went with the lad, my satchel full of medicines and bandages. We chatted together as we went along sharing, as opportunity came, something of the gospel.

After walking for nearly an hour we reached his home. The headman greeted me gruffly, his leg was sore and he was in much pain. He had managed to stop the bleeding and had then covered the long wound with cow dung. The sight and smell of it made me want to be sick, but I cleaned it and bandaged it. This took some time, but gave me the chance to speak of the power of Christ in overcoming the strength of the 'komun', which had such a grip on the people of that district.

Somehow I have never forgotten that scene. Two older men were with him, both completely naked and drunk. They grovelled in the muck of that homestead. Whenever I mentioned the name of Christ they sneered with satanic mockery and hate. But God honoured that visit and my halting words. The headman's leg was soon better and he became a great help later in encouraging boys to attend the school at Tamkal.[1]

It was through the schools' work in that area that the living church of Jesus began to grow.

Steady Progress

Although the intake each year since the end of World War II had not proved as great as had been earlier anticipated, yet each year a steady enrolment was maintained. In the 58th session (1960-61) 27 students enrolled including 9 missionaries who were on leave from their work abroad. This was a significant pointer to the continued need and value of the training the School gave.

At a time when inflation was virtually unknown, it is interesting to read in the annual report for that session of Sir John's appeal for supporters to consider subscribing to the funds of the School by means

---

[1] P.Price, God in the Valley (Patmos Press, 1970), p.15.

of a Deed of Covenant. He said, 'As the School is a charity we can reclaim tax on any amount given through a Deed of Covenant by a tax-payer who is resident in the United Kingdom and who pays income tax at the standard rate. Thus a gift of £2 plus reclaimed tax, becomes in fact a subscription of £3.5s.4d!'

It was an innovation in those days, but commonplace nowadays.

'Fellowship Day' 1962

The chill of a winter's morning failed to cool the enthusiasm of students committed to the task of making ready for this special day. With unity of purpose, preparations progressed. Slowly, the icy grip of winter relaxed and the sun shone in splendour as many friends gathered in the Boardroom of the Royal London Homoeopathic Hospital, where an atmosphere of happy expectation, imparted by the ever genial Chairmanship of Sir John Weir, prevailed. Mr R.I.Johnson OBE, was welcomed to give a lecture entitled 'Food Preservation - Past, Present and Future'.

With a subject close to the everyday needs of people, he at once engaged the attention of his audience, introducing them to biblical records, revealing the methods of food preservation used in the ancient world, and then advancing through the centuries, he told them of the present-day scientific and technical processes used.

After tea, the film 'Jungle Beach-head' exposed some of the cruelties of tribal customs practised by the early peoples of Viet Nam, which revealed the urgent need for their release from satanic power by means of the good news of the Lord Jesus Christ.

The evening session began with the Warden, Miss Bargh, presenting 'From Far Away,' bringing recent news of ex-students at work overseas, and so forging the links in the chain of fellowship embracing MSM students everywhere. This special greeting was sent to them *'Now may the God of hope fill you with all joy and peace in believing'* (Rom. 15:13).

The students of that year made their contribution by a novel interweaving of personal testimony into the narrative of an imaginary letter, whilst 'Introducing Kenya' was a feature of past student missionary activity given by Miss Muriel Holt serving with the Africa Inland Mission at Kapropita in Kenya.

Using the words of St Paul in 1 Thessalonians 2:8 *'...not the gospel ....only...but also our own souls...'* Mr L.T.Lyall, the guest speaker, stressed the obligation of missionaries not only to preach the gospel but also to give themselves without reserve as a requisite for reaching the people to whom they are sent.

'Half-a-Loaf' or a 'Slice of Bread'

'It used to be a favourite saying of the late Dr Edwin Neatby, that "Half-a-loaf is better than no bread at all!" He frequently used that expression in relation to the work of the MSM.' So said the President of the School, the Revd A. **Timothy Houghton** at the 1962 Annual Meeting. He went on to say,

> In these days it may be somewhat pretentious to call it 'half-a-loaf' as, of course, in one year's session students cannot learn half of what a doctor, or nurse, or a dispenser, or a dentist has to learn on their respective courses. Within a welfare state such as we in Britain enjoy, medical aid is freely available for everyone, but what is the position elsewhere in our world?
>
> Medical services in countries which are emerging as new and independent, if available at all, are in the main grossly inadequate to meet the need. Our missionary societies have done a magnificent work in attempting to fill the gap by treating thousands of sick folk, and in so doing they have shown in action, the compassionate love of Christ. But in spite of all this effort, the vast majority of people, especially in the villages and mountain reaches, are still in most cases without medical aid whatever, a factor which encourages them to seek the help of such local aids as witchdoctors.
>
> It is in this situation that the MSM, being unable to supply the 'whole loaf,' supplies that 'half loaf,' or even that 'slice of bread', which has been and is of such tremendous value. All over the world today there are missionaries who have felt that the knowledge and skill they received at the School has enabled them again and again to relieve human suffering and to tell many who are sick, of a Saviour's love, and who otherwise would not have heard.
>
> In thinking thus, one is reminded that these missionaries go out with not just 'half-a-loaf' or the 'slice of bread', for in the gospels we read how the Lord Jesus Christ went out and saw the five thousand who were hungry and in need of food. On enquiring as to their store, his disciples said 'There is a lad here with five barley loaves and two small fishes, but what are they among so many?'
>
> Maybe there are those today who are tempted to ask what is the use of sending out missionaries with only 'one slice of bread' to help meet the need, so vast as it is even today in many lands. But it should ever be remembered how the Lord *multiplied* those loaves and fishes, and the 5,000 were fed in abundance.
>
> Here is an apt analogy, for again and again men and women have gone forth from the Missionary School of Medicine making full use of

the knowledge they have been taught, but relying much more on the God on whom they depend, that He, in spite of their limited knowledge, has made use of their skill and multiplied it beyond all telling, to the benefit of thousands of people in dire need. To God be the glory!

So ended the President's comments at the conclusion of Fellowship Day 1962.

'The Diamonds'

Apparently, according to Mr Malcolm Hunter, the Monitor for the 1962-63 session, each year a member of the staff gave the student group a nickname, and because it was the sixtieth year they were designated 'The Diamonds'. At first, it was thought somewhat inappropiate by the student-body, but later they changed their minds and accepted that they were really *'Black Diamonds'* - another name, for coal! *Black diamonds have one purpose - to be burnt out, to give warmth, and to be spent for the benefit of others!* It was their desire that the lives of the students might be devoted in God's time to God's work, and that they might shine for his glory!

Malcolm, addressing those assembled for the Annual Prizegiving, went on to express to the Staff the warm thanks of the students, especially for the toleration shown towards their *enthusiasm*. As a group they had been deeply impressed by the effectiveness of Homoeotherapy, and they endeavoured many times to try out the cures (or otherwise) on each other, which made some demands! They had also caught the idea of beautifying No.2 Powis Place and much planning and paint went into the effort.

Impressions of a New Student

Another student of that group, **Patricia Sills** SRN, gives some of her impressions of her time at the School:

It was the first day of the second term. Some of us were newcomers (trained or semi-trained nurses). We felt strange, and we looked strange too - a pale, tired missionary just arrived from the field, a bright uniformed Salvation Army lass, a Lutheran Deaconess with twinkling eyes which were not hidden by her rather formidable habit and quaint cap. Conspicuous by their shyness were three fair, blushing girls from the Continent who completed the group.

The seven old timers gave us a friendly welcome into their midst. It was soon evident to us that *they* were an equally assorted bunch. There were two Brethren, mischievously teased by a hot Baptist, and a keen Methodist lady lay preacher! A Pentecostal Sister presided benignly over the proceedings. A mixed group we certainly were, gathered out from Finland, Switzerland, Germany, Nigeria, Australia, South Africa and Britain. This was no ordinary course we had come to! We were in for 'GMT' as well! (Good Missionary Training).

'O give thanks unto the LORD for He is good...let the redeemed of the LORD say so!' (Psalm 107:1-2). It was a day of prayer. We had turned aside from lectures, clinics and exams for a time of fellowship in praise and prayer. We had so much to praise God for, ...had He not gathered us into this fellowship? Here we had seen something of the goodness of the Lord and learned and experienced so many new things together.

Medicine, ...such a vast subject, and the time so limited. How inadequate we felt. 'But God.' Different personalities and backgrounds, but we were learning something of that togetherness in Christ. Yes, we had much to praise God for. But we had gathered to pray too. Past students, now scattered throughout the world, were remembered in prayer. We discussed, thought of, and prayed about the opportunity and potentiality of medical missionary work in this area. We were also reminded of the vast out-reach through the distribution of Christian literature. Days like these helped to unite this diverse assortment of students.

'...let them exalt him also in the assembly of the people...' (Psalm 107:32).

Our last day of the session: friends and relatives gathered for the Annual Meeting and Prize-giving. It was obvious by the variety of prize winners that there had not been a lack of competition among the students. The successful ones were applauded, and we all rejoiced with them.

Our desire was, however, that above all, He should be exalted in this assembly. We were young people gathered out of the lands by Him, equipped and enabled by Him, and were going forth to the lands of His choice for us, Laos, India, Bhutan, Pakistan, New Guinea, Aden, Ethiopia, Tanganyika, Nigeria and Brazil.

'Abundantly Worthwhile'

Perhaps, in some ways, especially numerically, the sixth decade of the MSM was somewhat disappointing. It had been felt by the Council that, after the War, large numbers of prospective missionary candidates would apply to do the course. This did not quite happen as during this time only a few over two hundred took advantage of the training provided.

However, let this part of the story conclude with the talk by **Raymond Guyatt** from Hong Kong, a former student of the School, given at the Sixtieth Annual Meeting.

Some years ago, an Army Nissen hut was erected to serve as a clinic for work amongst the refugees which crowd into Hong Kong, and during this time I had the privilege of sharing in the work of the clinic. Our patients, often in extreme poverty, come at the rate of between one to two-hundred every day. They come with a very wide variety of diseases. In addition to the ordinary kind of complaints, they have diseases like tuberculosis, leprosy, and a lot of worm infections, including a particular liver complaint peculiar to that part of the world. We also get patients who without doubt require dentistry, and casualties also abound. There are many cases of scalds and burns among children because parents go out to work and carelessly leave children at home with stoves unprotected and burning hot.

In the clinic, we use quite a variety of medicines and local applications, but one of the great difficulties we have to contend with is pure ignorance. For instance, grass, earth and tobacco was applied to a badly cut head. Ointments, which were meant to be applied had been eaten. Injections must be given and needles inserted always on the painful spot *because this is done by the Chinese medicine man!*

Homoeopathy has been used in the clinic to good effect. Bryonia and Phosphorus for coughs and chest diseases are given a good deal; Arnica for bumps and bruises, and Belladonna for a number of conditions; Silica has been useful in bad dental cases when we inspected incomplete removal of stumps, and Chamomilla is a wonder to many in babies' teething troubles.

But the purpose of the clinic is not only to help the people, though this would obviously be of great benefit, but to preach the everlasting gospel and we have seen very many people turn to the Lord, many of them never having heard of God's redeeming love before.

My closing words must be expressions of thanks on behalf of all past students for the tremendous debt we owe to the Missionary School of Medicine, and to one and all who contribute to its welfare. To our President and Council, the Staff, the Lecturers, and all who support the work, we can only say that it is all *'abundantly worthwhile'* and we give them our very sincere thanks indeed.

8 A Goodly Company

Unusual Help from a Former MSM Student

One day at the end of 1965, Mr D.V.Everitt MPS, the Pharmacist at the RLHH expressed his gratitude to mission workers in Peru for their help in the collection of venom from the snake *Lachesis Muta*. Without such assistance this particular raw material would not have become available to homoeopathy in its best form for all the potencies needed. Having ascertained that the Lachesis of Peru was the venom required, the co-operation of three missionaries was sought, one of whom was an ex-student of the MSM.

Some specially designed containers were sent out and after nearly a year's effort, on the very day the former student was to leave Peru for furlough, his national assistant shot a 9 foot specimen just as it was about to strike a child! Immediately the vials were laid out and the venom was expressed from the fangs and posted to London by air mail.

There was no difficulty about customs duty as the South American officials had affixed a label depicting a large skull and cross-bones in yellow and red on the outside of the parcel, with the words 'Snake venom - keep away from food'. This possibly explained its very speedy transit! The head and skin of the snake were verified by the Curator of Reptiles at the London Zoo, as being that of the true *Lachesis Muta* of a large adult size.

This happy conclusion - after so much patient waiting by these mission workers in Peru - gave much satisfaction to all concerned and when further supplies were forthcoming, they were offered and accepted by all the homoeopathic pharmacists around the world. Reference to the 'Materia Medica' show the chief indications for the use of this drug, but the very short and reliable pointers will be found under, 'Mental symptoms - *great loquacity, jealous, suspicious, religious insanity, derangement of the time sense, worse for sleep*'.

Retirement of Key Persons

For exactly half the life of the Missionary School of Medicine - 31 years to be precise - Miss Elizabeth J. Bargh had been the Warden and Secretary: a wonderful record. She held office throughout the Presidencies of the Revd A. Timothy Houghton, and before that of the Revd W.H.Aldis, when the difficulties of the war years were faced as the School, in spite of constant danger, continued its activities in central London.

Miss M.Iveson, her efficient helper on the administrative and secretarial side for 18 years, also left at the same time, having given the best years of her life to this work at the call of God.

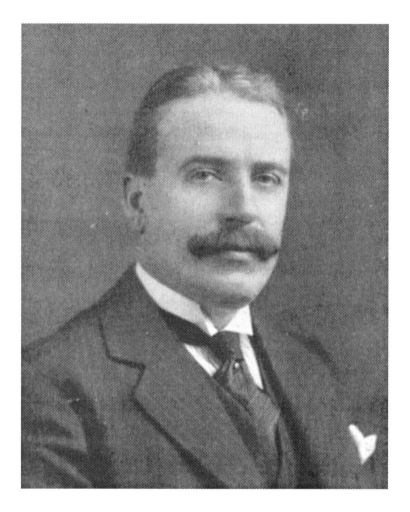

Sir John Weir

photographed, when as Dr. Weir he served between
the two world wars, as Chairman of the Medical Committee

At the end of the 1965 session, Sir John Weir retired as the Honorary Treasurer of the School, a post he had held since 1934, although his association with the MSM goes right back to almost its beginning. Among his many acts of generous kindness to the students, Sir John had regularly presented to every student at the Annual Meeting a set of 'Pointers to the Common Remedies' by Dr Margaret Tyler (consisting of about nine booklets), a most useful gift which was much appreciated by them all; the author of this history still has some of his! The reason Sir John took this step was because of his advancing years, although he agreed to continue to serve on the Council. He was pleased to accept the title of Honorary Treasurer Emeritus. His service was indeed outstanding and it would be true to say that the vitality of the School had been one of his major interests in the midst of a very busy life. Without doubt the School had been greatly honoured by his untiring support.

In her inimitable style, Miss Bargh wrote a Memorable Editorial in the Annual Report for 1965. It is worth quoting in full.

A Warden's Impression of Daily Life at the MSM and Beyond
What one may ask, *is* this Missionary School of Medicine?

Oh! its the place where the missionaries go to learn something of the missionary art!

The rendezvous is No.2 Powis Place, London WC1, just an old Georgian house not at all imposing, and many groups of students have been welcomed there. Usually they arrived with a great deal of curiosity and some trepidation but it was soon apparent that this quickly evaporated as they were introduced to one another and to those who were to be their teachers and friends.

No.2 soon developed signs and sounds foreign to other houses in the vicinity. From time to time Lecturers would be seen to come and go; groups of white-coated students, complete with stethoscopes and other medical implements, would sally forth from its portals on the way to hospital clinics and departments - a truly impressive sight! On their return, hunger predominating, large quantities of dietary concoctions would quickly disappear. Soon, peals of mirth would resound as an unsuspecting enthusiastic student endeavoured to hold forth on some obscure medical problem, being quite certain that he had solved it!

On certain days the Songs of Zion would be heard emanating from the Upper Room and many have paused as they passed along Powis Place. Alas, there were days when groans were heard! Examination days!

Many were the friends who helped during a session - quite wonderful: **Doctors and hospital sisters giving of their precious time and of their specialized knowledge, council members who take responsibility and guide the affairs of the School, business men, printers, photographers, electricians etc., porters at the RLHH who were indispensable friends, supporters and intercessors, so often unknown, and who gave of their time and strength and**

substance. A GOODLY COMPANY making an individual contribution to the well-being of all.

Days of training over, the time came to collect equipment and prepare and pack for the journey out, homoeopathic medicines must not be forgotten. Visas, permits, jabs, and 'what-not' are all needed as these young missionaries go forth to their God-given spheres and tasks overseas. There they labour, gaining an insight into the customs and needs of the people.

Many serve in hot and humid dispensaries in the tropical zones, some at leprosy centres, others serve by the wayside, maybe on trek, visiting villages with a mobile medical unit, or going by launch along dangerous waterways. A few have even ventured to the polar regions. But there they are, all intent in carrying out the great commission. A GOODLY COMPANY.

It can be said that over the course of years hundreds or even thousands of needy folk from every clime have benefited medically through the ministry of past students of the MSM and have heard and often received the glad news of a Saviour who loves and cares for them.

We rejoice that as a result of their service and witness there will be many among the 'great multitude that no man can number, of all nations and kindreds, and peoples and tongues, which stand before the throne and before the Lamb of God'.

It must have taken a while for the School to have recovered from the retirement of these three very key members of its Executive, but there was;

No Thought of Retirement at '65' for the MSM !

In 1968 the School reached the age of 65 years. The President commented,

By the analogy of reaching the retirement age and qualifying for pension, this might suggest that the School has now *completed* its working life, but we are happy to say that there is no thought of retirement for the School which continues to fulfil its purpose.

Numbers of students have never been large, and it is true that most medical missionary work has to be undertaken by skilled people who have qualified as doctors in medicine and surgery. But in spite of all the efforts of governments to step up state medical services, where in the past they relied on voluntary effort, it is still true to say that in the countries where missionaries are to be found there are vast numbers of people who would be deprived of any medical aid at all were they to rely only on what the state is able to offer.

Nor can mission hospitals, with their qualified staff, cope with any but those, often in overwhelming numbers, who can reach the hospital or clinic for treatment.

Evangelistic and pastoral missionaries, who are able to visit the villages, where the majority of people are to be found, can do an enormous amount to relieve human suffering on the spot, if they have the knowledge and skill that can be acquired by a course at the Missionary School of Medicine.

New Officers (and Some New Problems)

Taking the MSM into this period of post retirement were a number of new faces, the principle person being the new Warden and Secretary, Miss Lyle Bottom SRN,SCM,RST, who came to the School after a long experience of medical missionary work in India, as well as wide experience in hospitals in England, both as Sister-tutor and as Matron. Also, for a time during the post-war years she served as a visiting lecturer in Hygiene at the MSM.

Also, somewhat nervously, a new Honorary Treasurer took over from Sir John Weir. He was Mr Francis F. Stunt LLB, who wrote as follows shortly after taking office: 'I feel that I cannot bring to my duties quite the same enthusiasm, and certainly not the same sense of humour as characterized my predecessor during his Treasurership. He still continues to interest our friends in what we are doing and the gifts that continue to come in are most welcome.'

However, a change of financial officers was reflected in increased charges imposed upon the School for use of No.2 Powis Place. The new Treasurer went on to explain: 'For many years we have occupied premises in Hahnemann House, Powis Place, at a very moderate rental, and we have known that this could not continue much longer. Our rent is now much higher and indeed, almost every item of expenditure is rising. As will be seen from the accounts (1968), our income is insufficient to meet the expenses of the year's operation, in spite of the fact that our supporters gave more generously than in the previous year. In consequence we drew on our reserve fund which is mainly made up of gifts which have been intended to enable us to offer training at little or no cost to students. We are at present abating fees so that students are really only contributing about one-eighth of the cost of what the School provides for them. We are thankful that this is possible, but we depend upon the Lord's stewards for its continuance.'

A new Warden, a new Treasurer and also a new Physician to the Queen. This appointment was made public when it was announced that Dr M.G.Blackie MD, BS, MRCS, LRCP, Dean of the Faculty of

Homoeopathy at the Royal London Homoeopathic Hospital, had been made a Physician to the Queen in succession to Sir John Weir. Dr Blackie was a good friend of the MSM and had always taken an interest in its work, being a member of its teaching staff.

Teething Problems
Extracts from letters received from 18 ex-students working all over the world were printed in the 1969 Annual Report of the School. All of them spoke well of the way they were able to implement the teaching they received when at the School. One of them, **Bryn Jones** working in Brazil wrote:

> *'Will you come to our area to have a meeting?'*
> We assure the enquirer that we will make every effort to be there as soon as possible. Then comes the inevitable query, *'You will bring medicine and take out teeth won't you?'* or *'I can tell my friends who want their teeth out to come along, can't I?'*
> Very many come along to the meetings in the interior either because they have received medical help in the past, or because they want some.
> Dentistry is perhaps the part of the MSM course that has proved the most valuable. So many of the interior dwellers are in desperate need of dental treatment. Probably this is caused by the fact that drugs for almost any ailment can be bought from the local traders, whereas they are unable to extract teeth. Every part of the time at MSM has proved of value, but dentistry is particularly useful to a new missionary who can use it while still struggling to learn the language.

The day to day running of the School continued in much the same way as it had always functioned. Lectures were held each day together with practical clinical experiences. The students had some time to themselves for personal study. In her charming little book entitled, *SORRY....BUT...* **Frances Lyons** (née Linklater) writes vividly about one experience she had in practical dental training when a student at the School at this time.

> *'Did you get to any extractions today?'* was a familiar question asked by MSM students as two more unfortunates(?) arrived back from a practical at a London teaching hospital. After theory came the practical, and apparently, history had proved that if, through fear, and the consciousness of being only a novice, one refused to make use of a proffered opportunity, one never had a second chance.
> *'Yes.'* would come the excited reply.

'Well, what was it like? How did you feel?'

'Oh, I felt as I looked at the tooth between the forceps I was still clutching, that I had just climbed Mount Everest!' retorted one fortunate student.

My turn soon came. I arrived with my companion (we were always sent for our practicals in twos) at the entrance to the hospital. We were met by a rather abrupt and official-looking person.

'You two from the MSM?'

'Y..y..yes.' we stammered as we put on our white coats (regulation while doing practicals).

'Right, you', - pointing to my companion - *'go to outpatients, and you,'* - pointing to me - *'go down the passage, turn right, then left, take the lift to the second floor'* - or maybe it was the third - *'and Theatre is first right. You've to be with Sir...'*

Shall I ever forget that day?!

The operation had been a lengthy but fascinating one. The trainee dentists, who were all males, stood around the operating table. Theatre Sister was in complete control as only Theatre Sisters can be. Because of my short stature, I was allowed to stand right in front and next to the surgeon and, therefore, I was greatly privileged. I felt less so when the great man nudged me, and whispered from under his mask,

'You from the MSM?'

I answered in the affirmative. He brusquely, but not unkindly, ordered,

'Get scrubbed up.'

My! How I wished the floor could have given way under me, thus granting me a speedy exit! Remembering the advice of my colleagues, however, I obeyed. The cold perspiration which rained through fear from my brow had to be constantly wiped away by the rather irate Sister. It was one thing to perform such a menial task for a handsome young man, who, after all, was a trainee dentist, but having to do it for *this one*, well, it must have been hard for her. Although her reactions gave me anything but confidence, I did feel sorry for her.

'Ready?'

'Yes, Sir.' I replied, feeling anything but ready.

'Good, now remove the upper left molar.'

The atmosphere was tense, my hand shook, and so did the rest of me. I was also aware of a dozen pair of eyes peeping at me from the tops of their owners' masks, and I felt many a smile of amusement behind those masks!

I cried inwardly, *'Dear Lord, I can't do this. I am trusting YOU, for your glory is at stake here.'*

I struggled, and levered (one never pulls a tooth but levers) but that tooth would not budge. How glad I was that the patient was unconscious. My teacher, however, was encouraging.

'You are doing fine, keep at it; you've a good firm grip, you'll manage.'

Then it happened! I had reached my `Everest`!

'Well done.' said Sir... .[2]

MSM Ahead of its Time

The present day mood for mission expansion is coined best by the phrase 'Cross-Cultural' as nationals from one culture move across the world to witness to Jesus (and to learn of Jesus) in another culture. In the past, it was rather a case of 'The West evangelizing the Rest'. Thus it could be said that the MSM was ahead of its time as the seventh decade of the 20th century began, for the students entering the 67th Session were indeed 'From All Nations to All Nations', as after completing the course, students from Holland planned to go, God willing, to Asia, others from Tasmania to Gambia, others from South Africa to Nigeria, others again from Ireland to Brazil, and others from Finland to Ethiopia, and lastly, and perhaps more conventionally, some from England to Chad, and to the Yemen.

Adapting Courses

Owing to fewer students - characteristic of things to come - the Main Course lasting nine months gave way to shorter, more compact courses, that were of appeal also to other medical workers and missionaries on home leave.

Special visits were also arranged to the Renal Dyalysis Unit at the Royal Free Hospital, the Television Unit at the Moorfields Eye Hospital, and to a General Practitioner's Unit to see the modern Health Centre at Harlow New Town. The short special course in Tropical Diseases at the Wellcome Museum, arranged through the kindness of the Director, was of enormous value and twenty external students who were missionary candidates in training at different Bible Colleges were also able to attend these lectures. It was obvious from the way the various subjects were dealt with that a lot of preparation had gone into the Course which covered such topics as Cholera, Leishmaniasis, Snake-bite, Typhoid, Schistosomiasis, Leprosy, Malaria, Rabies and Helminthiasis.

---

[2]Francis Linklater-Lyons SORRY-BUT (Puritan Press Ltd., 1981)

Meanwhile, life continued to function more or less as normally, although with fewer students, the Warden had to use considerable initiative as the various adjustments were planned and worked out. Moreover, little by little new lecturers appeared, to take over from those who had laboured for many years; for instance, Dr J.Raiside retired from lecturing in Children's Diseases and he was succeeded by Dr. Anita Davies who carried on as a main MSM lecturer until the School ceased to give tuition in 1995.

Tragically, Dr. Raeside was killed shortly afterwards, together with thirteen distinguished people in the homoeopathic medical world, in an air disaster involving a Trident airliner en-route for Brussels. They were on their way to attend the International Homoeopathic League Congress in that city in 1972.

Post-Graduate Hazards of a 'Top Student'

Samuel Mattix left for Laos at the end of July 1972 after completing the full course at the School. He was 'Top Student' for his year. On the 28th October in the same year, the house where he was living with other young missionaries was raided by the Viet Cong and Sam, together with another young man was taken captive, two women missionaries being murdered in the raid.

Prayer was offered all over the Christian world, and on the 28th March 1973, five months from the day of capture, they were released along with other prisoners of war in Hanoi. Sam has since written the story of their experiences in the *Decision* magazine, and the following extracts were quoted in the School's Annual Report, by kind permission:

'The Blue Flower'
  During the 40 days on the trail to Hanoi, Lloyd and I did a lot of praying. Many times our prayers were directly answered. The sandals, for example, came just at the right time. At other times we would pray for a change of diet - for fruit - and it would come. Every day, we experienced His faithfulness for He would bring along food when it was most needed. One day my feet were really hurting and blisters were forming. The guard was setting a fast pace and I was limping along, my eyes on the trail, trying to keep up. Just off to the side I noticed a little blue flower .... I didn't have my glasses, (these had been taken away and Sam has bad eyesight) *but it looked like a Forget-me-not. I was blessed by seeing that little blue flower, because I realized that God had not forgotten me, that even then HE was with*

ME and HE CARED! It came at the right time and a reminder that all we are and have, comes from God.

Two verses from Hebrews 13 helped us greatly on the journey as captives, 'I will never leave thee, nor forsake thee.' The Lord is my helper, and I will not fear what man shall do unto me.' We had every reason to fear what man would do for us. Danger existed all the way, but we did not fear death.

Much of what we went through in those months of captivity proved profitable in prayer and meditation.

A Visit to Bible House

During the Spring term of 1972, the students were privileged to visit Bible House in London, where they received a copy of the Bible in the language of the country where they hoped to serve, providing of course, that it was available. There was the delight of exploring the spacous halls and illustrious library, and then viewing a missionary film. Their hearts were humbled as they saw the ancient manuscripts, and then the newest translation of the Bible into the Ketua language.

The time was so well spent and the students left Bible House, not only with a treasured gift to use in God's service but with a new zeal to be numbered with those who had gone before. The preserved writings both in ancient and new dialects stood as a witness that the work was not finished but still going on to its final completion.

A poem written by a student of the 1972 session, beautifully sums up how each MSM student experienced the Lord's hand upon their lives.

The Call

All has not ended yet - why, it's only the beginning,
  We're stepping out in Jesus' Name,
Good News of Christ we're bringing.
  We're bold and unafraid of man,
Of devils, death, or foe.
  For in God's power only
We all have dared to go.

'How can you go?' Some people ask,
    They are ignorant of their sin,
No need disturbs their child-like state,
    No need their souls to win.
How can we NOT GO our conscience cries,
    When Christ went all the way.
These reasons are but Satan's lies
    How can we - how dare we stay?
Rewards and prizes will be given.
    'Well done', we'll hear Christ say
As we offer the fruit of our labours
    On God's great Judgment Day.
When joy around the Saviour's Throne
    With those from every nation;
No colour bar, no rich man here,
    Not one from land or station.

All one in Christ whose blood was shed
    To redeem a world of sin,
The 'Call' has come to all our hearts,
    The CALL to SEEK to WIN.
How can we NOT go, our compassion cries,
    When its Jesus who sends us forth.
What is the price of a soul in gold.
    What to Christ - was one soul worth?

With this moving poem by Betty Clark we give God praise for 70 fulfilled years of the Missionary School of Medicine.

9 Medicine Serving Mission

With the advances in modern medicine and the general educational development of much of the 'Third World,' the need arose in the latter part of the 20th century for better qualified medical staff especially from indigenous populations. This meant that the kind of medical help given by those trained at the Missionary School of Medicine was becoming less needful. This was reflected in the falling numbers of those applying for training at that time. The world, however, is a large place and there were those areas then - as there are still - where skilled medical aid was scanty and where opportunity for such help as MSM trained personnel could provide, *was* still welcomed.   The Council of the School, therefore, *'did not lose heart'* (2 Corinthians 4:1) as they continued to plan for the eighth decade of its life.

Adaptibility
1974 saw the start of an experimental year which aimed to help those missionary candidates who could attend training only on a part-time basis, as well as continuing to provide for those able to attend the fulltime Diploma Course. This part-time facility was also of special benefit to those missionary students from the continent who were in London studying the English language. These represented many well-known international missionary societies whose aim was cross-cultural evangelism throughout the world.

Another small change reflecting this move of 'adaptability' was the combining of the Annual Meeting and Prize-giving in the afternoon of Saturday 22nd June 1974, with the Students' Fellowship Meeting in the evening. In chairing the afternoon session, the President, Canon A. Timothy Houghton, observed that it was exactly fifty years since he had completed his course at the School in 1924! Three students qualified for the full Diploma Course and six for the part-time Course.

The following year, yet another innovation was introduced in an attempt to attract more students to the School. This was to concentrate less on the 9 month course in favour of a shorter 3 month course. As a consequence of this major change the re-arrangement of the lecture programme still aimed to cover most of the subjects dealt with in the full course. This meant a greater reduction in practical work, but students were encouraged to stay on for another term for more practical experience. Obviously, this radical change in the lecture programme involved the Warden in a great deal of increased hard work which she bore without murmur in her own dedicated fashion.

Presidential Matters

The office of President has always been one of some importance in the life of the MSM, spiritually and administratively. From the beginning some very fine men of God have served the School in this office, inaugurated in 1906. The first was Captain James Cundy JP, a member of the Board of Management of the London Homoeopathic Hospital. Through him the School became closely associated with the Board. Captain Cundy was a member of the Council of the Church Mission Society. He passed away in 1911.

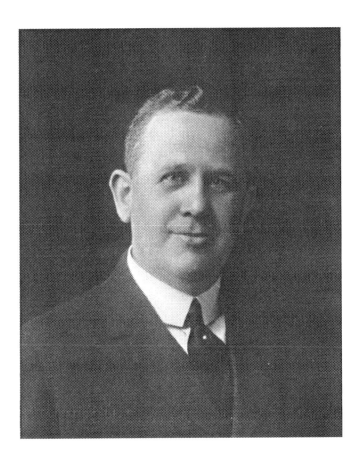

The Revd J. Stuart Holden, MA, DD,
President of the School

After a short interregnum, the Revd J. Stuart Holden MA,DD, accepted the post of President. At the time he was Vicar of St Paul's, Portman Square, London, a fashionable place of evangelicalism in the centre of the city, and he was widely known, here and abroad, as a convention speaker. He was also honorary Home Director of the China Inland Mission and he served the School with distinction until his sudden homecall in 1934. Dr Holden often told the students, *'You are touching the ends of the earth,'* as they went out by faith in obedience to their Master's command *'using Medicine in the Service of Mission'* .

Also associated with the CIM was the next President, the Revd W.H. Aldis, who served the School so faithfully for many years, including the difficult war years until his death in 1948. He was succeeded by the Revd A. Timothy Houghton, who features prominently in this history both as a student and as a pioneer missionary in Burma, serving with gracious efficiency for 29 years until 1977.

On Saturday18th March 1978, as many friends gathered for the Annual Meeting to celebrate the 75th anniversary of the founding of the School, minutes before it began, news was received of the sudden passing to Higher Service the previous night of the School's new President, Mr Len Moules, the General Secretary of the Worldwide Evangelisation Crusade. Canon Houghton unhesitatingly led the meeting, first in tribute and then on to praise, rejoicing that the Lord on high is King and that he rules over all.

After Mr Moules' sudden death, Mr Harold Dodd MB,ChM,FRCS was asked by the Council to be the next President. He first lectured in elementary surgery at the School in 1940 and then joined the Council in 1952. The author remembers attending Mr Dodd's lectures, as a student during the 50th Jubilee Session:

> As I recall the lectures given to us by Mr Dodd, I take down from my library shelves the book of notes which I took at the time. These notes travelled with me during the years following my time at the MSM and were especially useful to me in the remote area of NW Kenya where I served.
> Mr Dodd was probably in his prime in 1952. He was a tall man of slim build, alert, spritely, and a fine captivating lecturer. Although a top surgeon, he had the ability to relate the complexities of his profession to the possible situations his MSM students might encounter in the years to come. He covered such problems as injuries of all kinds, burns, abscesses, ulcers, infection, haemorrhages, wounds, fractures, etc. All

his notes, even now, seem to be so practical and helpful, covering both allopathic and homoeopathic treatments.

His particular emphasis, stressed in almost every lecture, was the importance of correct posture. Harold Dodd felt strongly that a multitude of ills and complaints could be avoided if folk could only learn and practise the importance of good posture!

Mr Dodd displayed at all times a fine Christian life and testimony. The words of Psalm 84:11 were really true of him: *'The Lord God is a sun and a shield, the Lord will give grace and glory: no good thing will he withhold from them that walk uprightly!'* Later, in his retirement, he was ordained into the ministry of the Church of England and served as a Non-Stipendiary Minister on the staff of All Souls' Langham Place, in the heart of London.

The Honorary Treasurer, Mr F.F.Stunt, who had been legal adviser to the School for many years was called to 'Higher Service' in 1977. He was a hard-working man who gave his all in a quiet unobtrusive manner. Mr Brian Weller, a godly and dedicated administrator, continues to serve as Honorary Treasurer to the present time.

The 'Student Body' in 1978-79
Listed below are the students who completed short courses during this Session. They are typical of each group in that their unity is measured, not so much in terms of their academic ability - as in most medical schools - but in their common desire, at the call of Christ to go into all the world to preach the gospel and heal the sick. The students in this Session were:

Angela Bailey MPS,
> a pharmacist from England, proceeding to Brazil with the Baptist Missionary Society.

Margaret Bartlett,
> a teacher from Australia who had already served for 14 years in the Solomon Islands.

Shirley Clewley,
> a secretary from Australia, hoping to work in SE Asia.

Peter Elks MA,
> from England, hoping to work with the Worldwide Evangelisation Crusade.

Lucy Holt,
> a teacher from England who had worked as an experienced independent missionary for 14 years in Bangladesh where she is now resident.

Anne Anderson,
> a civil servant from Scotland, proceeding to Brazil with the Unevangelised Fields Mission where she is still serving.

Evelyn Eglington BSc, PhD,
> from England, following in her father's footsteps as a missionary in Peru, associated with Echoes of Service.

Carla Hein,
> a linguist from the USA, proceeding to Indonesia with the New Tribes Mission.

Winny Koele,
> from Holland, hoping to work in India.

Pirkko Karjalainen,
> of Finland, hoping to work in SE Asia with Operation Mobilization.

Susan Peck MA,
> from the USA, going to Africa with the Wycliffe Bible Translators.

Stanley Potter,
> a Baptist minister from the USA serving in British Colombia with the Peace River Mission.

Mrs Marlene Sundermeier,
> of Germany, to Sri Lanka with the Kandy City Mission and later to South Africa.

Two of the above commented about the special mini-courses they attended during their time at the MSM. Dr **Evelyn Eglington** wrote:

> From October 23 to 27 the MSM students went into a Homoeopathic Retreat, being allowed to attend the intensive week of lectures in Homoeopathy held for doctors, by the Faculty of Homoeopathy, in the Boardroom of the RLHH. As Dean of the Faculty, Dr Margery Blackie chaired most of the meetings, and also gave a lecture on 'Pathological Prescribing in Rheumatism' on the final day.
>
> Many aspects of rheumatism and arthritis were considered: osteo-arthritis, chronic and early troubles, root-referred pain, the factors which aggravate the condition such as heat and cold, movement, etc., and the remedies indicated according to the patient and his symptoms. For those in General Practice there was an extremely helpful lecture by

Dr Jack about the introduction of Homoeopathy into the busy work of a GP, to the benefit of doctor, patient, and the National Health Service. In conclusion, the use of a Homoeopathic Repertory was demonstrated to show how best to decide on the indicated remedy for a particular patient.

In all, an interesting week, and helpful to our Homoeopathic thinking.

Miss **Carla Hein** reported on 'Paediatrics and Nutrition' at the Tropical Child Health Unit's Institute of Child Health. She wrote:

'Lo, children are a heritage from the Lord' (Psalm 127:3). This verse of scripture came to my mind often as I and the seven other students were able to attend the autumn course at the Institute of Child Health. We had our vision widened to the needs in nutrition and health care of the ever-increasing number of children in the developing countries, in the world round about us. But in turn we were presented with practical knowledge as to how we can help and teach those we go to, how disease and malnutrition may be decreased.

With 1979 being The International Year of the Child, we trust that with practical tools such as we have received, and the message of Christ we have to share, that many more children will be able to enjoy the health and life *we* have.

Effective yet Harmless
One of the major benefits of teaching Homoeopathy to prospective missionary lay people is that, unlike conventional medicine, if the wrong remedy is prescribed, it is unlikely to cause ill effects. This is because of the minute amount of the drug that is actually given. Dr Samuel Hahnemann, the founder of modern Homoeopathy, discovered by experience that if a soluble drug, such as a plant tincture, were put through repeated stages of dilution and vigorous shaking, the remedy developed greater powers of cure, and undesirable effects from the crude drug were abolished.' (Quoted from *Essentials of Homoeopathic Prescribing* by Dr H. Fergie Woods MD, MRCS.)

In the use of Homoeopathy, there is no such thing as the undesirable feature of 'side effects' which sometimes occur when Allopathic (conventional) drugs are used, often resulting in more annoyance than the actual symptom itself. This is the reason why it is exceedingly unwise for unqualified people to prescribe conventional medicine.

Students at the MSM were instructed to gain a clear 'symptom picture' of a considerable number of Homoeopathic remedies so that when such were encountered in their varied fields abroad they would know which remedy to use. The author recalls an incident in his own experience when living with his wife and two very young children in a remote area in Kenya.

Having just returned there from a day-long safari to the nearest town to replenish supplies, our youngest child developed an acute and distressing fever. Her symptoms were quite alarming, flushed face, burning hot skin, rapid pulse with a high temperature, worse for lying down and seeming to wake into a delirium, tossing and restless. We were very anxious and resorted to prayer. The thought of returning the 70 miles through mountainous country which we had travelled the day before was anything but attractive. Then we remembered Belladonna! The symptom picture seemed to match perfectly. A few granules of that drug were given and we soon noticed a dramatic improvement. It was a gracious answer to our prayers.

Margaret Bartlett's experience was similar. She had worked as a missionary teacher for many years before joining the 1978-79 MSM course. She wrote of her faith in Homoeopathy in this way:

> Homoeopathy came into my hand early in my missionary experience. Dr Northcote Deck of the South Seas Evangelical Mission in the British Solomon Islands had introduced 36 Homoeopathic medicines which he thought would cover the needs of the people there. I was fortunate enough to have his excellent knowledge handed down to me. This encouraged me to treat people by matching the patients' symptoms with the proven remedy. It was not long before I began to see people respond. Fevers abated, 'whoops' ceased, bruises failed to appear, fractures were helped, and many of the common ills responded to this unfailing LAW, when rightly applied. Of course the remedy could be wrong and so no help was given. It meant trying again and again, and looking to the Lord for wisdom.
>
> Then one unforgettable day I was challenged to take over a small hospital while the nurse tried to escape for furlough. The day before, she said to me, 'There are some very strange symptoms presenting themselves at the clinic, in fact they are frightful!' Then, early the following morning, her last words rang out as the ship left a realistic gulf between us - 'Oh, if you think it might be poliomyelitis, try GELSEMIUM!'
>
> And so, this little insignificant 'Yellow Jasmine' in the hands of the great Hahnemann became the remedy for the hour of epidemic in the Solomons. People came by canoe, by foot, by day, by night, ceaselessly for many weeks. Some were hospitalised but many lay helpless in the villages awaiting medication. A pattern seemed to emerge. If they took this medicine in the 30th potency within half-a-day of first feeling the

symptoms, they would recover, even though for some there was a period of suffering and extreme weakness.

Out of this experience I personally became an ardent advocate of Homoeopathy. I studied each case. I proved God! I stumbled on remedies for my own fever, for obstinate bronchitis. I longed to do the Missionary School of Medicine course which included Homoeopathy, but 12,000 miles was a long way from the School. A retiring missionary bequeathed her 'Materia Medica' to me, and, most of all, I began to build up my own list of case histories.

The year 1978 has been a challenge for me, and a joy. My wish regarding the Missionary School of Medicine has become a reality. I know so little but I have learnt so much. My present burden is *Homoeopathy for Missions* and the Lord of the Harvest is the One I completely trust to lead me in His paths and teach me for future ministry.

Under Law?

Mention should have been made before of a somewhat severe letter each student was given on the first day of a new course. Perhaps it reflected the kind of culture in London when it was first written, but looking back now at the beginning of a new Millennium it does rather seem as though the Warden and Council members thought of the students as rather wild juveniles! At least we all knew where we stood. The letter read as follows:

Rules for Students

Students are required to attend REGULARLY and PUNCTUALLY and to sign the register morning and afternoon. For the work of this School REGULARITY and DILIGENCE are of more value than brilliance. This will count towards prize-giving. Students will get out of the training, in usefulness, confidence and power, what they put into it in careful thought and study.

The LECTURERS and CLINICAL TEACHERS are voluntarily giving time and trouble to enable students to acquire the elements of medicine and surgery for use in their work in isolated districts in foreign countries. THEY must not be disturbed by late-comers. TEACHERS are occasionally liable to be late, being unavoidably detained, but students should await their arrival unless notified that they are not coming.

The work of this School must take precedence over other work, meetings, etc. Speaking appointments must be at a minimum. The giving of time and energy necessary would not be fair to students or School. Students must be present at all lectures and fixtures unless given special exemption.

LIBRARY

Books may be borrowed from the Library. Two books can be taken away by each student, but must be returned at the end of two weeks. Will students enter their names and the title of the book in the 'Library Book'. The Library is in the charge of two Librarians, and they will need your help and co-operation. The Study Room is available and SILENCE there is desirable. Students working together on any subject may converse in a low voice not to disturb others.

Well now, we kept these instructions most dutifully. **But we all had great fun!**

The Warden goes to Texas

Lyle Bottom, the Warden of MSM, was invited to go to the USA in the summer of 1979 as a guest lecturer to help initiate an 'Emergency Medical Course' at Christ for the Nations Institute at Dallas in the state of Texas. This was the Warden's first visit to America and she found the experience very rewarding. After her return she wrote:

> Christ for the Nations Institute in Dallas has 17 buildings in 40 acres, with accommodation for 1,400 students, whose ages vary considerably and who augment their income by doing outside work in their free hours. Courses are offered in Bible Training, Languages, Music, Singing, Radio and Television Production, Deaf Ministries, and Flight Training. The vision of the Institute is 'World-wide Mission'. I was able to give lectures in Tropical Hygiene, Malnutrition and Paediatrics, Emergency Obstetrics, and Homoeopathy. I made many new friends and contacts. The outreach from the Institute is vast and I was able to attend various lectures of deep interest. Although every day was full I was able to include a visit to the Wycliffe Translators International Headquarters in Dallas, and the well-known Baylor Hospital, seeing a service in operation which is so widely different to that in England. There was also an opportunity to be interviewed on Television Channel 39 on a Sunday programme, to speak of the work of the Missionary School of Medicine.

Small and Beautiful

From the immensity of Christ for the Nations Institute in Dallas, the Warden returned to find just 16 students waiting to begin the 76th session. This was one of the new Short Courses covering three months intensive medical training - the 6th to date - and the candidates came from many different countries. Although covering quite a wide syllabus for so brief a course, the main work was on Homoeopathy and students were encouraged to know the leading indications of fifty remedies.

More changes were soon on the way both in personnel and in daily routines. In the 1980 course the pattern of instruction at the School was significantly altered, partly because the premises at No.2 had to be shared with the Faculty of Homoeopathy who organized intensive post-graduate courses in Homoeopathy for qualified doctors. MSM students had the privilege of attending some of these lectures. Formal lectures at the School were greatly reduced in favour of concentrated tuition at the Wellcome Museum of Medical Science for Tropical Diseases, and the Tropical Child Health Unit for paediatrics, and nutrition. Students were also encouraged to take the Certificate for First Aid set by the St John Ambulance Association. A bonus for the students was that as this instruction was given at the City of London Centre, the certificates were duly presented at the Mansion House by the Lord Mayor of London in his ceremonial robes.

Other outside hospitals continued to open their doors to students for instruction in casualty departments - Poplar Hospital, Hackney Hospital, Bethnal Green Hospital, General Lying-in Hospital, and the Dreadnought Seamen's Hospital. Eye instruction was also given to students at the Moorfields Eye Hospital.

Dentistry was always high on the agenda and all over the world, past students have been grateful for the instruction they received. For many years Mr N.E.Gillham LDS,RCS, taught the students, but with dental facilities no longer available at the RLHH, although retired by 1980, he came a long distance to give theoretical tuition.

Mr J.N.Le Rossignol FCHS, also retired after 40 years at the RLHH where MSM students had attended his clinics in Chiropody. Mary Skinner, a former student, wrote from Ecuador: 'Yesterday, I extracted my first Quachua-Indian tooth! I counted the roots and they were all intact. It is amazing too, the kind of shoes our American and Canadian colleagues wear. Just the kind that keeps one busy. But these folks can now walk in comfort thanks to Mr Le Rossignol's teaching on Foot Care.'

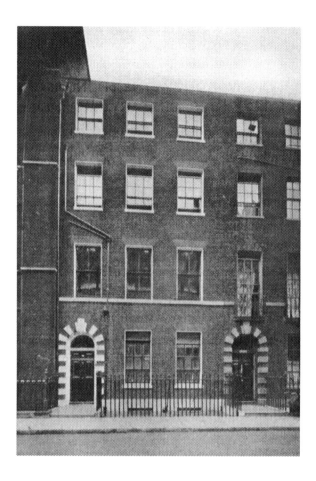

No.2 Powis Place
Adjacent to the RLHH

Into the Eighties
'Number two' Powis Place, the long time home of the Missionary
School of Medicine, is one of a small number of properties situated in
a cul-de-sac off the famous Great Ormond Street, London. Powis Place
was once the site of the first Powys House which we are reminded was
built in the reign of William III by William Herbert, Marquis of Powys
and prior to its demolition in 1777 wheresported a water reservoir on
the roof stocked with fish for angling purposes!

On the corner of Great Ormond Street and Queen's Square, was the
house where Lord Macauley lived and where, with Wilberforce, he

carried on an unwearied crusade struggling against the slave trade: an outstanding achievement in the history of the nations.

With such associations, No.2 Powis Place was a fitting location for an institution with the aims and motivation of the MSM.

Against the background of world conditions at the end of the 1970s, scientific and medical progress and the changing pattern of missionary work, MSM completed more than seventy-five years and experienced 'the hand of God that doest wonders' (Psalm 77:14). He is the master of all circumstances, multiplying our 'little' and making it his 'much,' giving wisdom and grace for all our problems. Staff changes were always a recurring challenge and at the beginning of 1980 another milestone was reached in the retirement for health reasons of both the Head of Studies/Secretary, and of the President.

Miss Lyle Bottom SRN,SCM,RNT, served the School after the retirement of Elizabeth Bargh. Prior to her appointment she had worked in India for 18 years in medical service with the BCMS (now known as Crosslinks) and with ZBMM (now called Interserve). During that time she was awarded the Kaiser-i-Hind medal for her contribution to nursing training in India. She also held a number of important posts under the NHS in England, as Sister Tutor, and finally as Matron of the War Memorial Hospital in Carshalton. She came to the MSM expecting to give ten years service but she carried on for fifteen, standing the test of changing circumstances and needs, resulting in the abandonment of the full 9 month course in favour of a more intensive 3 month course.

Canon Houghton wrote of her at the time of her retirement in this way: 'I always found Lyle, not only professionally competent but eager to maintain the spiritual standards which the School has always set. Her students, of many nationalities, greatly loved her and found in her a helpful guide in their studies and one, who on the personal level, had a sympathetic understanding of their problems.'

In the goodness of God Mrs Jean Hayward-Lynch SRN,SCM, was appointed deputy to Lyle Bottom at the beginning of the 76th session and was able to start under her instruction and assist in the management of the autumn short course, so when Miss Bottom became so seriously ill - for the first time in her 15 years of service at the School - Jean was able to take over the full running of the School and was appointed the new Head of Studies and Secretary following Lyle Bottom's retirement. Miss Bottom, after her recovery, continued to serve on the Council until her death in the early nineties.

Unexpected Miracles

Emily Rowntree, who was a student in 1948, came back to the School thirty years later to do a refresher course. She had worked during all those years in Angola and recalled some of her experiences:

> I left for Angola shortly after taking the course in 1948, a place not known to many, and as one Portuguese trader described where we lived, as 'beyond the moon', it seemed to me to be indeed at the ends of the earth! Communications were poor and irregular, and indeed, continue so, as we have just been over three months without mail! Supplies have also been irregular but one has been most grateful to the Lord for a knowledge of Homoeopathy. On many occasions we would have had to close our hospital had we not been practising Homoeopathy, as no other drugs were available.
>
> We run two small hospitals, one at Cazambo, where we live, and the other at Cavungo thirty miles away, where five nurses do regular clinics. We had well over 500 babies born here last year, and our normal clinics can be for anything from 500 to 900 patients. Naturally, we have seen many good cures and quick ones too, treating babies with measles, whooping cough, diarrhoea, fevers etc.
>
> One notable case, was a man who had had a stroke and spent several months in hospitals. He was unable to turn in his bed, and indeed, I was not anxious to start treatment when others had failed, but his wife begged us to. He was a Christian: so with Baryta Carb, Gelsemium and Curare, within a month he was sitting outside on a chair, and shortly after, walking. He lived for years on a dose of Curare at irregular intervals and kept in good health. This is only one of the miracles I didn't expect!
>
> Many patients travel hundreds of miles to have treatment where we are and often leave the government hospital for some of our 'little sugar pills'. Every patient receives Homoeopathy and we find it a great help as an addition to the conventional medicines for Tuberculosis. It is a great privilege since last September to be able to take a few months at the MSM again. It has been a refresher course in many ways, again meeting many lecturers who have been so faithful in teaching all down the years. May the Lord bless them richly in return. Their help has been so invaluable to so many of us working in isolated areas - 'Their labour is not in vain in the Lord'.

10 God Makes No Mistakes

A New Team

After serving as a medical consultant at the RLHH for many years, Dr Kathleen Priestman MRCS, LRCP, FF Hom., was a familiar figure to MSM students as they attended her clinics, where she treated them with the utmost courtesy and respect. She explained the different cases with much care, often in language which was not too technical. As the students sat there resplendent in their white coats and with stethoscopes at the ready, normally highly nervous, she had the knack of putting them at ease, even including them in her consultation as she discussed the necessary treatment. It was therefore, not all that surprising, when she assumed the role of President at the commencement of the 78th session.

As Dr Priestman began her period of office she wrote:

> On the mission field nowadays there is a much greater emphasis involving training members of the indigenous churches in very simple methods of diagnosis and treatment, as a means of combating disease, malnutrition and ignorance and of showing the love of Christ in action, which, they say, speaks louder than words.
>
> A few of the most frequently used homoeopathic remedies and a knowledge of how to use them, must surely add an even greater potential to the value of the simple medical boxes provided, but someone must teach this knowledge to the indigenous Christians and someone must teach the expatriate missionaries. The courses at the MSM are planned to fulfil this need, and the Council would like to feel that they were more widely known and used by Missionary Societies.

At the start of this session, only two students had enrolled on the courses! A strenuous effort was made in advertising the MSM facilities to various training colleges and missionary societies but sadly, with little response. However, an advertisement in the Christian youth magazine *Buzz* resulted in a mass of enquiries from all over Britain, so that for the second short course there were six students present. Due also to financial cutbacks, the Royal London Homoeopathic Hospital had to close the operating theatre and a number of surgical wards, which meant a limitation of some training facilities previously available to the students.

Meanwhile, the new Secretary and Head of Studies at the School, Jean Hayward-Lynch, tackled her new responsibilities with determination.

She had a unique link with former MSM students in that she had done her nursing training at the RLHH, during which time she was ill and also became a patient there. The prognosis was discouraging, and wondering if it would be possible for her to continue with her call to missionary service overseas, she later wrote:

> I shared my sorrow with the MSM students, and oh, how we prayed! From then on I did recover, so I feel I owe a real debt to those students. During those training days, Lyle Bottom was our Sister Tutor in the Preliminary Training School, and as we both loved the Lord, we warmed to each other. Over the years we kept in touch, especially when I was on furlough from Zambia where I was so privileged to serve for 20 years.

> As I face this new task of working as Warden of MSM, I marvel at the way the Lord has led me in preparation for this great work - I did office and accountancy work when I first left school; I was a nurse, I had had the experience of being overseas; I had been Editor of the Zambian Nurses Christian Fellowship magazine; I was a great organiser of others! Something I did not really take as an attribute, *but God makes no mistakes!*

Yet Another Testimony

During 1981, **Barry Haigh**, a student at MSM during the 1964-65 session wrote about his experiences:

> When I was a student at MSM I thoroughly enjoyed every minute of it, even though it was very hard work and not much time for eating meals during the week. Sometimes I wondered if all the hard work would be useful and I can say without hesitation that it has. Firstly, for myself personally, especially when I was a bachelor and living alone, it was a help to know if I was seriously ill, or just neurotic. Then, when I became a family man with a wife and two boys, over and over again I have been able to prevent an illness becoming serious or know when to rush off to the doctor, which is a very long way from where we live, over awful roads which are often impassable anyway. Secondly, it has been invaluable as a means of both showing mercy and getting to know personally the African people of this area. I am able to share more fully in their lives, joys and sorrows. One area I didn't expect to get involved in was their marital problems. We virtually have a marriage guidance clinic here now.

> To preach the Gospel alone is insufficient, we must *do* also. Let me give you an example. When I was first learning the difficult Lunda language, I was preaching the Gospel but not very effectively, stumbling along. One old lady was not listening too well and I thought maybe it was because I was stuttering, but I found out later that she had

a terrible toothache: a wisdom tooth with an abscess. So I offered to extract it. As soon as I put the forceps on it she began to howl with great volume. I noticed it getting dark around me and looked up to find a great crowd had gathered to see the 'white man' murder the African woman! That made me very nervous and together with her howling I was almost sorry I had offered. Suddenly, to my relief, the tooth came out in one piece to the applause of the crowd. Next day, I noticed two things. She listened when I preached. It hadn't been my poor Lunda at all that was preventing her from listening, and secondly, a lot more people had toothache also.

That was the start of a clinic which I had not really wanted, though I feel it is a golden opportunity for the Lord. There is no other medical facility in this area despite modern government policy to be fully responsible for their medical care. The country just cannot keep pace with the already existing clinics. It is a joy to me to know, without being too boastful, that there are many people alive today - some new believers in Christ - who would not be alive but for my medical help.

For any prospective missionary going to a country such as Zambia and away from a city, I would strongly advise that not only would the MSM be useful, but essential!

A Renewed Threat to Homoeopathy

As the School approached its 80th anniversary it found itself in increasing contention with those who discredited Homoeopathy for one reason or another. Sadly, some parts of the Christian world at that time joined in this criticism, accusing Homoeopathy of being saturated in the 'occult'. Dr Kathleen Priestman, rigorously defended Homoeopathy, speaking from a lifelong experience of its effectiveness in all her professional work. Writing in the Annual Reports for 1982 and 1983 she said:

> The Missionary School of Medicine is in its 80th year. Many students and many people from all over the world testify to its worth, so it has been sad to have Homoeopathy accused of being occult in the Christian press in 1983 - a false accusation.
>
> Samuel Hahnemann was a qualified chemist and physician, very concerned about the treatment of sick people, people as individuals, as whole people. As a chemist he was interested in the effect of drugs and experimented on himself using quinine, which was used successfully in the treatment of intermittent fever. He found that he developed a 'rigidity of joints, numbness and aching of all the bones of the body and a kind of stupefaction of the senses,' all symptoms associated with intermittent fever, which lasted some hours after taking each dose and recurred every time he repeated a dose and not otherwise.

Friends confirmed his findings and Hahnemann started testing - 'proving' he called it, - other substances used in medicine at that time. He found that they produced the symptoms in his 'provers' that they were finding in their treatment of sick individuals.

This resulted in the basis of Homoeopathic treatment. The patient is treated as a whole person, as an individual, and the remedy which will help them most is the one where the symptoms produced in healthy 'provers' most closely resemble the presenting symptom complex of the sick person.

Hahnemann was concerned that the medicines should be used in the smallest effective dose, surely the best way? And although this has led to high dilutions known as 'potencies,' the succession seems to increase their clinical effect.

It appears that Hahnemann's use of the expression 'vital force' is his attempt to explain the mode of action of Homoeopathically prepared medicine in the human body. However, his use of dilute remedies, and that he was a Freemason, and that later in his life he sometimes used mesmerism, are the main reasons why Homoeopathy is said to be occult and Christian people told to avoid it. This seems about as unreasonable as to say that a Christian should never play a musical instrument or listen to an orchestra because Tubal, a direct descendant of Cain, was 'the father of all such as handle the harp and organ'! It should also be remembered that Mozart was a Freemason but we all love his music.

I have used Homoeopathic medicines all my professional life, and feel sure there is no connection with the occult. I acknowledge Jesus Christ as my Saviour and my Lord.

As the Missionary School of Medicine goes forward into the future I am sure that God will continue to bless the students as they seek to use what they learn, including Homoeopathy, in His service all over the world.

Another testimony in the defence of Homoeopathy came from a qualified nurse, almost at the same time as that of Dr Priestman. **Jenny Hearne** who attended the School to learn about Homoeopathy wrote:

As a trained nurse I was all the more aware of my need to be further equipped and thus I commenced the MSM course without even knowing the basic principles of Homoeopathy - that the most successful remedy for treating and curing the ill, is that which produces the same symptoms in someone who is well. This was indeed a new world! A welcome one, too, since my nursing experience had left me with great reservations concerning conventional drug treatment, largely because of toxic side effects. In fact, I had a basic suspicion of anything in tablet form, so it was quite a task that lay before the lecturers to convince me of the validity of Homoeopathy. How quickly I was won over! The concepts of the whole person being considered in formulating treatment, and also the lack of toxic side effects, were new, exciting and very reassuring, as was the theory that Homoeopathic treatment stimulates the body's own immune system to fight disease. I began to feel positive instead of negative about Homoeopathic medication as a form of treatment.

Our teaching took the balanced form of lectures, written work, and attendance at outpatient clinics. There was hardly time to eat, especially on a Tuesday, but how we all looked forward to our lunch-time lecture with Dr R.W.Davey, whose humour and expertise enabled us to comprehend and enjoy this new and complex subject; truly one of the highlights of the week was to walk through the streets of London, to his consulting rooms. The written work, set for us weekly by Dr Kathleen Priestman, was designed to make us think 'Homoeopathically' and work things out for ourselves - a very valuable exercise. Attendance at the outpatient clinics at the RLHH, gave us the opportunity to see the theory working out in practice. How encouraging it was to see the patients being relieved or cured of conditions for which conventional treatment held little hope.

These three components of teaching were so ably supported by Mrs Hayward-Lynch, who did much to confirm and amplify our grasp of the subject. As my husband and I await the Lord's leading, for future service abroad, we are finding opportunities for practising this 'new world' of Homoeopathy - on ourselves! Minor accidents and virus symptoms have been dealt with very successfully, and we rejoice in God's promise to equip us in every way needful, for this work and sacrifice.

A Modest Increase in Students

Everyone in the School and on the Council were encouraged by an increase in the numbers of students during the early eighties. At times they wished they had elasticated walls at No.2 as the place was simply bubbling with activity again. It seemed a great answer to the prayers of many. Did it mean that more folk were becoming burdened about the needs of the world?

The January to March session experienced particular difficulty when snow was persistent, and industrial strikes seemed to go on and on, but as a group of God's children at MSM they were able to say, with Paul, that in whatsoever state they found themselves to be they were content.

Only on one day, when there was a complete shut down of the London Transport system were students and other personnel of the School and Hospital not able to attend lectures or clinics. At all other times, during those days, lecturers were at the School on time and some gave even more than usual.

To the list of teaching staff at that time, was added the name of Mr Stephen Bazlington, a dental surgeon with experience of overseas service in Ethiopia. As a child brought up on Homoeopathy, he spent quite a long time in the RLHH as a patient. His lectures were colourful and full of information about dentistry; sometimes the students wondered if he ever stopped to take a breath!

New equipment was purchased and new brochures printed and every effort was made to keep the School as up-to-date as possible. During the early part of the summer a number of Bible colleges were visited in order to speak of the School and the specialist training it offered. As a result, some students applied and were accepted.

The rooms at 2 Powis Place leased from the Trustees of Hahnemann House were freshly painted - almost as a celebration of 80 years since the Missionary School of Medicine was founded - the colour scheme chosen was quite dazzling and bright, turquoise with emerald green doors from bottom to top, reminding those who used them of the glory of God's creation with much beauty and colour. The Secretary and Head of Studies reflected on those 80 years as she wrote in the Annual Report of that Session.

> The Autumn term ended with a *Christmas at Home* on the 14th December when a very happy time was spent by all. Refreshments were served as the people arrived and then the students took it upon themselves to enact some of the lessons they had learned during the course which can best be described in the poem they wrote and recited:
>
> Ivan was there and now he's here, 'St Vincent is my home'
> But England, for the last 12 years has been a place to roam.
>
> Next from Finland, Palvi 'I've been a nurse two years'
> Helping with children back at home, trying to calm their fears.
>
> And Paula who's from Portugal, 'Angola too before'
> I'm going back to Bible School to study even more.
>
> Elsa was from Australia, here for so short a stay
> Her painful back became much worse, and so she left one day.
>
> And Ruth from England, 'I'm the one for ever asking "Why?"'
> So you can learn to understand that these my friends soon learned to sigh.

God Makes No Mistakes

We've studied many different things, read books both old and new,
We've taken notes in lecture times, and answered questions too.
A weekly test devised by Jean ensured we learned each part
Connected with anatomy, lungs, kidneys, liver, heart.
She taught us how to give a jab, in just the perfect place
And how to give an enema with courtesy and grace.
Gordon, our Red Cross friend and guide, came weekly with his cases
'Inflatable Annie' there inside, to put us through our paces.
'Give four short breaths' our Gordon cried, we all tried hard to obey
But ended in just laughing, so Annie died that day!
The subject that for all of us was, oh, so strange and new
Was that of Homoeopathy - we hadn't got a clue.
Our grey cells got an awful shock to learn such lofty things
The potencies, modalities and remedies and things!

11 Drought And Downpours

In Retrospect

At the beginning of this history, as the reader may recall, two subjects were compared with each other, both having occurred in 1903. These were: the first flight in a man-made aircraft, which lasted less than a minute, and the first steps taken by Dr George Burford and others who were physicians at the London Homoeopathic Hospital towards the foundation of the Missionary School of Medicine. In the following eighty years, enormous development took place in these two realms of aeronautical achievement and medical treatment. So far as the former was concerned, two world wars brought significant strides in the design and production of sophisticated aircraft. By 1983, air travel had improved beyond recognition and fast, safe and comfortable journeys to all parts of the globe made travel for missionaries considerably easier.

Similarly, all around the world, even in many of the developing countries, great progress was made in those eighty years in the treatment of sickness and disease. The principles which lay at the heart of the training offered at the MSM, whilst still valid in 1983, were however, less urgent because of the vast improvements in the training of indigenous medically qualified workers and the establishment of hospitals and health centres in so many parts of the world. Hence a missionary proceeding in that year to many remote areas, on becoming ill could usually find medical help available at a clinic within reasonable reach. Of course this was not so everywhere, but generally speaking, such was the case.

Difficulties in Student Recruitment

Partly for this reason, during the ninth decade of its history the recruitment of students became increasingly difficult. Although Council members spent a considerable amount of time seeking to rectify this situation, as will appear, it was all to little effect.

Inevitably, another problem the School faced was the logistics of managing these rather specialized training courses due to the low numbers of students, coupled with the uncertainty from term to term as to whether there would be *any students at all*. In 1950, the Faculty of the School numbered 38 highly qualified professionals who gave their services almost entirely free of charge; in 1984, this number had fallen to just 13. Thus more and more responsibility fell upon the Warden who shouldered the burden of extra teaching duties as well as handling all the administrative tasks.

Dr Kathleen Priestman, the School's President, writing in the annual report for 1984, had these and other matters in mind as she wrote:

> What is the role of the Missionary School of Medicine in today's world? A world where National Governments are taking increasing responsibility for the physical well-being, and National Churches the spiritual well-being of their peoples. This is reflected in the greater difficulty in obtaining visas for missionaries in many countries.
>
> At the same time there seems to be a decreasing interest in missionary work amongst young people in this country. Fewer and fewer candidates are offering for service abroad. The number of students for our courses this past year, five in January and only two in September, means that the School is running at a loss financially, in spite of the necessary increase in fees, which may have also contributed to the small number of students.

In point of fact, at the beginning of the September term the Warden was expecting seven students to do the course. All the necessary arrangements were in place, lecturers notified and ready to teach, plans laid for a smooth course. *Then, only two students turned up!*

A Striking Contrast

In stark contrast to events at MSM during 1984 was the talk given at the Annual Meeting and Prize Giving at the end of that year. The speaker was **Raymond Lower** who was on home leave from his work in Nagoya, Japan. He said:

> I came to the Missionary School of Medicine in September 1946 upon being demobilized at the end of the last war. Miss Bargh, who was then the Head of Studies, had a most gracious firmness in controlling, what was I believe, *the largest intake of students ever received at the School*. Looking at a photo of our year, all gathered with 'Charlie' the skeleton in the Anatomy classes, reminds me of the hilarity, yet depth of Christian fellowship and sense of vocation of our large group emerging from the war years. We had the privilege of a few lectures from Sir John Weir, the King's physician. I remember the insights given us in the Homoeopathic lectures from Dr Wheeler in the Boardroom of the Hospital; the humour of Dr Quinton as he lectured on Diseases. I remember too the adventures in our outpatients' clinics, the paratrooper who fainted as I stitched up his hand; my consternation when I did not have time to extract the second tooth as the patient was coming round from the gas!

After leaving the MSM Raymond sailed with his fiancee to China. As they were not yet married, the custom was in those days for couples to remain single until some knowledge of the language was acquired and they were sent to different locations some seventy miles apart. As things worked out they had only one year in China, virtually the whole of which was spent in language study. Raymond was proud of his dental achievements which he attributed to his MSM training:

> I can remember several occasions when I was able to help people in much pain from decaying teeth. I received one of the MSM dental prizes and I thought I was rather good at this but did not have enough of the Chinese language to find out what the patients thought!
>
> I remember one 'miracle' cure when a boy came with his head full of oozing sores. I was baffled, but on his second visit diagnosed it as an utterly neglected case of ringworm. I made up and applied a carbolic acid ointment which gave a rapid cure.

They had to leave China in 1950 when most overseas workers were expelled and were posted to Hongkong where they were allowed to marry. Shortly afterwards they were sent to Japan, where they commenced language study all over again! In Japan, which had a very good medical and dental service, a person was not allowed to practise medicine or dentistry without being officially qualified; however, Raymond was able to help friends on a number of occasions with suitable homoeopathic remedies.

His wife had contracted malaria whilst in China, and although the disease was not prevalent in Japan, she continued to suffer from malarial symptoms at regular intervals. She was greatly helped with the homoeopathic remedy 'Cinchona China'. They were also able to use homoeopathic remedies very effectively with their own children and never had to call a doctor except on two occasions, when bones were broken. Raymond Lower concluded his talk as follows:

> Looking at the spiritual work, which is of course the centre and goal of all missionary endeavour, I believe that the homoeopathic principle of looking at the patient as a 'whole person', rather than as a 'body' with something that has gone wrong, is vitally important. To whatever country one goes, human beings come under the Biblical description of having spirit, soul and body. The spirit of man is never satisfied until finding the reality of true fellowship with God. I can clearly remember the comment of an elderly Japanese gentleman, who after reading the Bible for the very first time said, 'You know, this really makes sense. I have worshipped and prayed at many a temple and shrine, but deep down inside me I have never had a sense of having made contact with the creator God. One who not only made everything, but who controls

it all, and has a plan for everything to fit into.' A year later he found fellowship with God through Jesus Christ whom he received as his Saviour.

Throughout the remaining years of the 'eighties' the MSM continued to *struggle to survive!* In the Annual Report for 1990 Dr. Kathleen Priestman wrote:

'The Missionary School of Medicine might be said to have been - like Elijah - in a *state of drought* for these past few years, with decreasing numbers of students and a dwindling income. Yet how wonderfully God has provided - just like in Elijah's day - He has provided students, however small their number, and legacies to maintain our resources...'

Signs of a 'Downpour'

Actually, the records show that the School had more students in 1990 than in the previous ten years. There were ten students in all - seven for the January to April course, and three in the September to December one. They were certainly an 'international' bunch, representing the USA, Britain, Holland, Finland, Switzerland, New Zealand and Germany. Four were going overseas with Operation Mobilisation, one independently with a Christian Brethren background, two with Worldwide Evangelisation Crusade, one with New Tribes Mission and two self-supporting.

Also in 1990 a new initiative was introduced for a limited period, just one day a week covering Tropical Health and Homoeopathy. Although at first attendance was disapponting, eventually two students became regular with another eight from the Abbey School in Central London where many Christians from overseas worked at improving their English before going to the 'Mission Field'.

A Change of Image

Frequently during the years of the late eighties the Council of the School gave very serious condideration to finding ways of making the MSM more appealing to those for whom it was originally founded, namely missionaries preparing to serve overseas. It was felt that perhaps the image of the School had become outdated both at home and in those countries where Christian missionaries were becoming much less welcome. To remedy this it was decided to consider a change of name for the School, to re-design the badge, to revise the Constitution and possibly to prepare a more attractive brochure. These changes involved much prayer, discussion, thought and planning, all undertaken in a voluntary capacity by members of the Council.

So far as the change of name was concerned, it was strongly felt that the well-known initials - MSM - should be retained. Various ideas were forthcoming such as the 'Neatby School of Medicine' (NSM - nearly there!) in memory of one of the School's honoured founders, but it was the Honorary Treasurer's suggestion which finally won the day - MEDICAL SERVICE MINISTRIES.

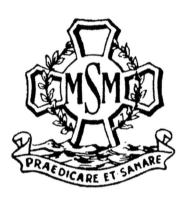

The enthusiasm of the Council members was then directed to the badge itself. The original one had summed up the principles of the School with such graphic simplicity (Motto, World, MSM, the Cross, Healing leaves) yet it seemed somewhat dated, even Victorian! Various designs were proposed and eventually the experience of Graham Turner, a professional artist, was sought. He came up with the final solution - so clear and positive, with very distinct features covering the famous initials, the motto, the world, and for those who are looking for it, the making of a Cross.

Another member of the Council, Ray Dadswell, gave dedicated attention to the revision of the prospectus and when it was finally accepted the main problem - can you believe it - involved what colour to use as a good background! Again members were consulted and they eventually agreed on the strong medium blue which made it so clear and distinctive.

The Constitution of the School, last reviewed in 1978, was also revised and printed in such a way as to conform with the 'new look' stationery. Very minor amendments were recorded and, for the first time, the EMA (Evangelical Missionary Alliance, which today operates under the title, 'Global Connections') Statement of Faith incorporated in full.

Another plan was to commission a video of the School's work and daily routines. Eventually, however, the whole idea was scrapped as proving both too expensive and too difficult to implement.

In the first term of the 1990 Autumn session a new experiment was tried where each week, and just for one whole week, all the lectures were devoted to only one subject, such as Anatomy or Homoeopathy, rather than a little of each, week by week. This had the advantage of appealing more to students who might join the course mid-term. Fortunately, those responsible for lecturing agreed to make this proposal work if it would make the whole structure of courses more appealing and practical to future student intakes.

Problems at Number 2

Meanwhile accommodation at No.2 was proving somewhat difficult. In the earlier years of the School, distinguished medical persons who carried great weight at the London Homoeopathic Hospital did all they could to grant every kind of practical help in the use of almost the whole of 2 Powis Place for the School at the most modest of rental terms.

Sadly, as these patrons passed on, the premises were taken over more and more by the Faculty of Homoeopathy, so these highly valued privileges were diminished and in 1990, the School was confined to using the top floor alone, and at times even this was under threat. Rental charges also became heavier and heavier. The Secretary and Head of Studies often sensed an almost resentful attitude on the part of other users of the building. This she found difficult to cope with, especially when the day to day oversight of in-house services fell to her. At one point the MSM was without gas for four months.

If the School was to continue into the future, it was becoming obvious to the Council that other accommodation - at an even higher rental - would need to be considered.

The Annual Barbican Fayre

Each year during this time, Dr Anita Davies and Dr Evelyn Eglington, both lecturers and members of Council, held a stall at the May annual London Barbican Fayre, for the purpose of raising funds for the School. The receipt of a cheque for £100 from the organizers was warmly welcomed by the Council and thanks were extended to these two good friends for their annual labours.

A New Publication

Mention has already been made of the suspicion felt in some evangelical circles regarding the authenticity of Homoeopathy as a valid Christian method of treatment. Fortunately, a member of the Council, Ronald Male MPS, had written a comprehensive statement called *The Bible and Homoeopathy* which he described as 'A defence of Purist Homoeopathic Medicine'. The Council agreed in 1989 to print 1,000 copies of this booklet for sale at £1 a copy with all proceeds, at the request of the author, donated to MSM funds. Athough availability of this booklet was advertised in a limited way in the Christian press and many copies were subsequently sold and widely distributed, as we go to press this title can still be supplied.

More Downpours

It seemed a strange fact, that during a period when the School was 'experiencing drought' due mainly to the shortage of students, *money in the form of some substantial legacies* continued to be given. This supply from the Lord's servants of a past generation continually made the Council wonder what the future role of the MSM was to be. At the end of 1989 cash balances available for the School's use amounted to £35,027.56 and the balance sheet total of funds was in excess of £80,000. Such a happy situation was due largely to the receipt of a legacy from the estate of Mr S.F.H.Butcher, whose wife predeceased him and who left no children. Mr Butcher had died in 1982, and after payment of nine bequests the residuary estate was subsequently divided equally between two parties. MSM being one of the two. Another even larger legacy, shared among several beneficiaries, was received from the Executors of Daisy, Lady Ogle.

The Hon Treasurer, Brian Weller, however, wrote a strong word of caution at the time to all Council members:

> It is marvellous how the Lord sustains the work of the School and while we do and should rejoice in His provision, one wonders where to draw the line. It is all very well to say 'The Lord will provide,' but as responsible officers it falls to us to take responsibility for balancing the books and providing for the continuation of the work of the School.
> We cannot expect legacies to cover the excess of expenditure year in and year out simply because this has been our experience during the

last four years. There must be either a concerted effort to increase gift income or some scheme of cost saving. One would be loath to raise fees above the present level of £500 for a non-residential course...

A New Vision Needed?

Suddenly, and at a time when the School faced so many difficulties, the Missionary School of Medicine found it had more money in its reserve than perhaps for the whole of its previous history. Was God leading the Council to think in terms of a new and different vision? This was a question the Council had to resolve, although, as we shall see, there was not total unanimity about the matter.

12 All Change

Presidential Change

Upon becoming an octogenarian, Dr Kathleen Priestman felt it was time for her to retire as President of the School. She had begun teaching at the MSM when she was just twenty-five years of age. Kathleen had occupied the post of President since 1981, thus her contribution to the School must be considered as outstanding. She will long be remembered for her quiet unassuming manner and her wise judgment and advice on a multitude of issues during what were quite difficult years for the MSM through the late eighties.

Dr Priestman presided at her final Council meeting as President on 11th March 1991 in the presence of Mr Alfred Lodge who had agreed to assume her duties as the new President. Thanks were warmly extended to the retiring President and her family for 'the lovely Christmas spread that was put on at the end of the autumn term' at the 'Christmas at Home' event in her Crowborough home.

Dr Kathleen Priestman welcomed Miss Mavis Knowles as a member of Council and Mr Alfred Lodge as the new President 'from this day on'. A word of thanks was given to her for all her years of service to the School. As a token of appreciation a cheque for £250 was presented to Dr. Priestman. This was for her new television set, which was needed and 'already much enjoyed!'

In presenting the Honorary Treasurer's report, Mr Brian Weller tabled draft accounts and sought the opinion of the Council regarding fee charges for future 'missionary' candidates should the School extend its facilities to 'Commercial Christians' who might consider taking the course.

Mrs Hayward-Lynch gave her report on the current details concerning the School. One student unexpectedly returned to the USA as she found the culture shock more than she could bear! This left three students - all living at the Foreign Missions' Club - and all were missionaries on home leave. New lockers, for student use, had been delivered, and the session was going well.

The need for a new sign at the front entrance to No.2 with the new name of 'MEDICAL SERVICE MINISTRIES' was discussed and Mr Weller said he would look into it.

Mr Lodge closed the meeting with a reading applicable to Dr Kathleen Priestman's leaving, and a prayer.

Ardent Zeal and a Sudden 'Homecall'

The new President of the School, was a man of great enthusiasm: just the sort of personality the School needed at this crucial time in its history. Mention of Alfred Lodge has already been made in this account. What enthusiasm he displayed when enrolling as a student at the outset of the Second World War when he arrived at Queen's Square on a bicycle having cycled from his home in Yorkshire. He subsequently served the Lord with his wife for many years in Nigeria working in association with CMML, travelling there for the first time in convoy for safety from enemy action on a voyage fraught with many hazards, but kept in safety by the Lord's good hand.

Armed with all the 'New Look' literature of the MSM, so recently and attractively produced, Alfred Lodge made it his business to visit many Bible Colleges and Missionary Training Institutes all over the country speaking about the facilities the MSM offered to missionary recruits proceeding abroad at the call of the Master. However, Alfred was not as young as he had been when he made that epic journey from Yorkshire to London in 1939. He presided over the Annual Meeting of the School in 1991 but very sadly, shortly after, suffered a severe heart attack from which he did not recover.

Warning Signs

In spite of all the efforts made by Council members in these recent years, the fortunes of the School did nothing but decline. The Warden, Jean Hayward-Lynch reported to the first meeting of the Council in 1992 that, 'To date there are no applicants for this year!' Dr Kathleen Priestman, still a member of Council, voiced her feelings after this notice from the Warden -

'As there was no sign of any students for the present year and the fact that Mr Lodge in his short term as President was so fervent in making the work of the MSM known and then was taken so suddenly from us, should we not take this as a sign from the Lord that the time had come to wind down?'

Vigorous discussion followed, which seemed to concentrate more upon the need to enlarge the Council than search for students! However, eventually a 'fairly' unanimous decision was reached that the School, should go forward in faith, praying for *five new students to apply for the May and October courses*, believing this would be a sign from the Lord to labour on. Some members of the Council were of the opinion that a Public Relations (PR) Assistant should be appointed to work alongside the Warden to facilitate a wider understanding of the School's work throughout the nation. One or two names were suggested to be approached for this work. A Job Description was in mind and some suggestions sent to the Warden.

However, the Council eventually approached Trident Public Relations Limited to audit the activities and goals of the MSM and to give further advice as appropiate.

Meanwhile - on a more mundane level - the lease for use of the rooms at No.2 Powis Place expired at the end of 1992. The Council were therefore forced to face the alternatives of either applying to the Hahnemann House Trustees to request an extension or to seek alternative accommodation in the RLHH which might well have cost as much as £13,000 per annum!

Upheaval - Without and Within

One of 1991's most unforgettable events, so far as the School was concerned and which affected the smooth running of its activities day by day, was the massive reconstruction work undertaken at the Hospital for Sick Children in Great Ormond Street, much of which was just across the road in Powis Place where the MSM was situated at the famous Number Two.

At the same time, the interior of No.2 was redecorated from top to bottom. These changes prompted the Secretary to write in the Annual Report:

> To both students and lecturers over this period, I would like to apologise for all the inconvenience and occasional headaches. Inside Hahnemann House (No.2) after the decorators left us, the all-white look at first seemed rather stark but we have come to appreciate this as it gives a fresh appearance and the house looks more spacious. For those of you who have trundled up and down stairs for lectures, you will be surprised to hear that there is no Lecture Room as such now. Our present position at the top of the house was known to many of you as the 'Museum' and to others as the 'Common Room' and even to others as the 'Quiet Room'. These are now my office, and a 'Common-cum-Lecture Room' with a small clinical room. We are still thankful to have the use of the kitchen on the second floor.
>
> I would like to take this opportunity to thank all the personnel at University College Hospital A & E Department, Guy's Hospital Dental Department and the Royal London Homoeopathic Hospital Clinicians for the time and help given to the students. We never fail to hear from the students how much they appreciate the kindness and the many

valuable things they learn. We have had a few new lecturers this term and we thank them all for the skills and time given to MSM and our thanks go to all the lecturers who have been coming so faithfully to teach our students over many years. Especially, I would like to mention Miss Mavis Knowles, a retired lecturer from the London Hospital and a one time missionary in Zambia, for all the help she gives to our students both in teaching and with practical advice.

Student Appreciation

Fiona Haines, a student at MSM during that period expressed her gratitude to the School as follows:

My time at the MSM was short but memorable. I attended on the Tropical Medicine Study days once a week in the Autumn of 1989. The knowledge gained on a variety of aspects of Disease and Health Care was obviously very useful. But the course gave more to us by introducing us to resources available from AHRTAG (Appropriate Health Resources and Technologies Action Group) and ECHO (Equipment to Charity Hospitals Overseas).

For me, however, the highlights of the Course were the lectures on Homoeopathy and the visit to Ainsworth's Homoeopathic Pharmacy - to be able to *see* the preparations being produced and learn about 'the how, the when, and the why' was fascinating. As someone who has benefited from being treated with these medicines, it completed the picture. I shall be going overseas well equipped and prepared with my case of homoeopathic remedies.

The Head of Studies Sums Up

Reporting on the 1992 session, Jean Hayward-Lynch wrote very graphically:

I am pleased to say the building projects going on around us here in Powis Place, continue with a lot less noise, or is it that we get used to all the banging and drilling?! However, the cracks in the office ceiling are certainly larger and the dust comes crumbling through everyday. With only one room now available for lectures and recreation for the students, we are constantly trying to ring the changes. Sometimes we have desks and chairs, another time we try sitting around a large table. The kitchen is used more as a rest room these days and it is good to take a short journey downstairs for a change of scenery.

Last June, we had five nurses come for one week mainly to study Tropical Diseases, but along with this came requests for dentistry, anaesthetics, all in one week! Can you imagine it? We were indeed stressed, both nurses and tutors. If the subjects are what they feel they *need* for the *area to which they are going* we are only too pleased to help. Most of these nurses are with refugee agencies, with the same desire as a missionary to reach people with the Gospel. During the Autumn term we were able to help two nurses; one stayed a week, the other for two. It really is a joy to see these workers lap up all the information available in the short time they can donate to such valuable preparation.

We were privileged to have Pat Harman come and lecture on 'Nutrition and Child Care'. For many years Pat worked at the Child Health Institute alongside Professor David Morley. We do thank Pat for coming and making valuable contributions to the course, despite her busy schedule.

The highlight once again this year is Dentistry. The visit to Guy's Dental School is so enjoyed by our male students and I would like to take this occasion to thank Mr Pinkerton who arranges the clinics there and even contacts me when he thinks the students have not attended, when in fact they were already there!

The least enjoyed hour of the week is the weekly test paper time. We do feel this is important so that we can gauge whether or not the subject matter taught during the previous week has actually been absorbed or not. Recently, I have been reading a report of the year 1979 commenting that because the courses have reduced from nine months to twelve weeks they will need to become much more intensive. As the years have gone by I feel we have, perhaps, become a little too lenient, so I plan doing something about this.

Each term finds us visiting the Appropriate Health Resources & Technology Action Group which provides information and an enquiry service for health workers in developing countries. We also visit Equipment to Charity Hospitals Overseas. Here again we are able to purchase instruments, equipment and medical materials at a very low cost. Some buy a lot knowing what they will need for the future, others just browse, but it helps them greatly to know of these resource centres. On another afternoon we visit the Human Biology Section of the Natural History Museum in Kensington. This is relevant and useful, helping the students to gain a good knowledge of Anatomy. Thanks to Miss Knowles, they get a good all round knowledge. In fact the students often ask for more, which unfortunately, time does not permit in such a full programme. However, we do encourage students to read various books, giving 'chapter and verse' as it were, for their evening homework.

Travelling doesn't get easier for any of us. We cover our journeys with prayer, not only for safety and protection but for opportunity to witness for the Lord. One has only to look around at the faces of those travelling alongside us to see how unhappy many appear to be. We in

fact had one young lady from America here who designed a tract for us
to use on the Underground, with a smiling face on the front with
appropriate verse and words.

We share our joys and sorrows, for many are separated during these
weeks from wife or husband, children and close family connections.
Last year one student left her husband at home to care for four of their
children! We thank God our Heavenly Father, that He is always with us
to care for us.

A Time to Laugh
It was the great theologian Karl Barth who emphasized that eternity is
unrelated to time - when we die, we move outside the realm of time. In
recent times the civilized world in particular has been dominated by the
importance of 'not wasting time' leading to enormous stress, especially
in the work place as workers are required to fit more and more into the
time available. What wisdom there is then in these words from the
book of Ecclesiastes -

There is a time for everything, and a season for every activity
under heaven:
a time to be born and a time to die,
a time to plant and a time to uproot,
a time to kill and a time to heal,
a time to tear down and a time to build,
a time to weep and a time to laugh, ... (3:1-4).

It is possible that, whilst we recognize the Lord's goodness to the
School over the years of its existence, it would seem that throughout
the 1980s and beyond there was sometimes more cause for 'weeping'
than anything else. So much effort and planning went into the
organization of the courses and amenities offered by the School yet so
often there seemed to be fewer and fewer students wanting to do the
course. All quite depressing?

1993, however, gave all those concerned the joy of 'a time to laugh'!
To begin with, the School gained a new President, after being without
one for a couple of years. The Revd T.Omri Jenkins responded to the
invitation sent to him at the beginning of the year. He was a most godly
person of 'senior years' who had been much involved in mission,
mainly with the European Missionary Fellowship and through the
London Theological Seminary, and the Council greatly looked forward
to working under his leadership. Writing in the Annual Report for 1993
he said:

'My first year as President of the MSM has been an education for me. Having known of its good work over many years, I now see how little I knew of the devotion and effort of those responsible for organising its affairs and teaching students. Nothing is more gratifying to them, and to all who help MSM in various ways, than to know that so many missionaries and Christian workers are now using their training among the world's needy peoples.'

Then there were -

Two Anniversaries

Jean Hayward-Lynch, the hard working Head of Studies and Secretary, celebrated in 1993 forty years of being associated with the MSM. She recalled how in 1953 when she was a nursing student at the RLHH attending the fiftieth celebration meeting of the School, when there were 25 students doing a year's course, the writer of this History being one of them, she wrote:

'Little did I know at that time how the Lord would later call me back from medical mission work in Zambia where I was serving with Echoes of Service. For 40 years, God prepared Moses in the wilderness to undertake a special work for Him, and without my years in Africa, I do not think I could have taken over from Lyle Bottom as Head of Studies. The Lord God has been so gracious during all those years. Abundant or lean years, no matter. He makes us glad. The standard of our work in His Name may have varied over so long a period, but still He is pleased to look upon us with favour and to prosper our weak efforts.'

So it was that the MSM celebrated its 90th anniversary on 20th November 1993.

What an occasion that was!

For many months the members of Council had been planning the activities. A commemorative Souvenir Programme took many weeks to put together. Special features were discussed and implemented by the Council. It was a pleasure to hold the event in the Westminster Chapel made famous by the ministry of great expository preaching by such men as Dr Campbell Morgan and Dr Martyn Lloyd Jones, himself a medical practitioner favourably disposed to Homoeopathy. For this occasion the School valued the permission to use this famous venue given by the Rev R.T.Kendall, the presiding Minister.

The London Emmanuel Choir - known throughout the UK - was present and gave a superb programme of suitable choral music, their President, Mrs Muriel Shepherd, a long supporter of MSM spoke words of encouragement from her heart to all present.

Two past students of the School, **Elizabeth Flemming** and David Ryan, spoke of the value their training had been to them. Miss Flemming had worked as a missionary nurse in Sierra Leone. She acknowledged that while MSM had prepared her for many of the things encountered there, the smells and sights and noises which assailed her on arrival were something of a shock. The range of tasks which she tackled in the Lord's strength revealed her strength of character and pioneer qualities. **David Ryan** talked about his work in Brazil and testified to the help and care he was able to minister while visiting village communities. As a result because of what he had learned at the MSM he was much sought after by those suffering sickness and injury.

Many former students attended the event, some from as far afield as Germany, Holland, Ireland, Scotland and Wales.

Dr Anita Davies ably assisted by ladies attending Westminster Chapel provided good refreshments and a birthday cake with 90 candles to mark the occasion. Many were the greetings exchanged and opportunities to renew acquaintances while the displays and literature provided further items of interest.

A Fine Testimony to the Value of MSM Training
Included in the Souvenir Programme, available free of cost at this 90th Birthday celebration, was a testimony from **Sue Frampton** to the beneficial work of the Missionary School of Medicine. Sue had worked with the WEC in Ghana after completing a course at the MSM.

'The MSM course was the most useful thing I have ever done. The majority of lecturers had practised abroad in primitive conditions and they prepared us well for work in a developing country.

In Ghana, for three-and-a-half years, I had been unexpectedly thrust into the role of 'doctor' because I knew more than any of the local people, and undertook the MSM course during my first Home-leave. My two fellow pupils on the course had both received medical training and had served in their home countries, one as an anaesthetist in Korea, and the other as a psychologist in Bolivia. We all got on extremely well, boarding at the Foreign Missions' Club in Highbury.

The course covered an amazing amount. The full timetable, with numerous modules, often included late sessions as when we did microscopy at the Tropical Diseases Hospital, and resuscitation at St Bartholomew's. Evening study was needed in order to keep up with the course. The facilities made available to us at the Institute of Child Health were particularly helpful. Here are my impressions of the course syllabus-

ANATOMY   I achieved a good understanding of the various body
    systems, quite enough for what I needed.
NURSING   One of the most useful parts of the course. It was so
    practical: taking temperatures, sterilizing instruments, tube
    feeding, enemas, stomach wash-outs, suturing, giving
    anaesthetics and injections, removing foreign bodies, care of
    burns including grafting, all with a little sized doll to practise
    on!
MEDICINE AND DIAGNOSTICS   We were taught how to take a
    history of a case, and observe, and diagnose in the absence of
    modern laboratory facilities, so relevant to Ghana.
TROPICAL   Not a lot of this was new to me, but for a first-time
    missionary, invaluable.
DENTISTRY   We had several lectures and about four days at
    Guy's Hospital Dentistry Department watching extractions
    and local anaesthetics. Dentistry is simply not available at all
    in any of the local hospitals in Ghana, so I am in great
    demand. I also do a lot of oral hygiene with little children,
    saving teeth and preventing serious, disfiguring diseases.
ENVIRONMENTAL HYGIENE and CHILD HEALTH   Covered
    basic primary health care, looking at the causes of ill-health
    in the developing world and how to pass on this knowledge to
    the local people. We studied the growth and development of
    children, immunization and childhood diseases.
EYE DISEASES   We learned how to identify problems requiring
    expert attention but also many useful basic procedures.
FIRST AID   This included resuscitation in addition to the treatment
    of burns, bone fractures, and bleeding, supplemented by visits
    to the University Hospital Outpatients Department.
OBSTETRICS   We were taught the norms of pregnancy and
    childbirth as well as how to deal with emergencies, which is
    actually all one is usually asked to help with! This is an area I
    feel the most lack in and have since accompanied an

independent midwife on her rounds. Even so, my limited knowledge has proved useful in Ghana on several occasions.

HOMOEOPATHY   This was completely new to me and I was sceptical at first. However, I have found my limited knowledge of the subject very useful and have been impressed with how well it works when you get it right! I have successfully treated infected wounds which did not respond to penicillin tablets, a retained placenta, after-birth pains, burns, chickenpox to name a few.

My knowledge is quite sought after by my fellow missionaries as well as by my family and the local people.

It is two years since I was at MSM, so I may have left things out but this gives you an outline. Advice is given on what books, charts and medical assessories to acquire and how to obtain them with guidance on securing the best terms.

By the time I last left Ghana I was seeing 45 to 50 people a day, seven days a week, quite confidently and amazed by what I was able to do and the success rate. Literally dozens of children's lives have been saved and the people love us as a result.

I do not believe there is any better way to show the love of God in action to needy people. It is often the case that in the remote national hospitals the treatment is appallingly bad with some personnel caring little if the patient lives or dies, especially if the patient is from a less prestigous tribe. In contrast, they know I have loved and cared for them and always did my best. They know too that our God cares and helps and I can only give Him all the credit and glory, with sincere thanks to everyone who taught me at the MSM'.

How we must praise the Lord for all the 'Sue Framptons' - well over 1500 of them since the School began in 1903 - who have gone forth from No.2 Powis Place to **'preach and heal'**!

Indeed, '.. a Time to Laugh!'

The Thanksgiving Appeal
This special appeal for the Scholarship Fund was launched at the 90th Birthday gathering. From its inception the MSM had been dependent upon voluntary contributions and bequests. It had never been financially supported by student fees alone, nor had there ever been adequate endowment funds. A Bursary Fund existed to provide for the abatement of certain student fees by up to 25% but even so there was

awareness that increasing interest in MSM courses from *overseas candidates from the Third World* was being disappointed because many were unable to contemplate the expense involved in 10 weeks tuition and board in London.

The Thanksgiving Appeal was intended to fund the course cost in full for those who otherwise would have been unable to benefit from MSM training. In faith the Council looked to God to cover the cost of at least ten students a year. Donations of £1,000 or more were designed to produce annual interest and the smaller gifts treated as immediately available for approved Scholarship applicants.

At the end of September 1998, the response to this appeal had reached £20,133. Incredible!

Public Relations Manual

It will be recalled that in its desperation to make MSM more widely known the Council had approached a Public Relations company to audit the activities and goals of MSM. At considerable cost, and after an even longer period, this company submitted its report in November 1993. The Manual was in many ways a major disappointment and generally speaking only stated what was already largely known. Eventually, it had to be faced by the Council, that 'the writing was on the wall' for the MSM and it could not continue *in the way it had for 90 years under God'' most gracious hand.*

The time had come for 'ALL CHANGE'!

13 A New Ministry For A New Millennium

An Encouraging Conclusion?

As preparations began to formulate the changes being considered by the Council the School had a surprisingly successful year in 1994. For one thing there was quite an increase in numbers attending the courses and for the first time in several years students applied for the Spring session. Nurses attended the summer Tropical Medicine course and there were five enrolments for the Autumn term.

The video library also was steadily growing, thanks to Mavis Knowles and Richard Hayward-Lynch, who watched weekly for any television programmes that were suitable for teaching purposes. Several requests were received during the year from mission workers overseas who had particular needs and the Secretary and others were always ready to help. One nurse in Accra, with Wycliffe Bible Translators, found she needed to put her nursing skills into practice earlier than expected. The method of sterilisation by pressure cooker, which the School taught, had been forgotten. Consequently, she rang her father who got in touch with the Secretary who was then able to fax it on to his daughter. Another wrote from Ghana to say, that following the birth of a baby daughter, both she and the baby were ill with malaria. She felt it necessary to buy a microscope in order to use the knowledge she had previously gained at MSM, but sadly her notes on the subject were at home in Germany. The School was able to come to her rescue and provide a book on the subject.

At the Annual General Meeting, the two students who had just completed their MSM training were presented with their certificates and each gave a word of testimony. Janet White was the 100th student to be enrolled by the Secretary and Head of Studies, Mrs Jean Hayward-Lynch, during her time at the School. That enrolment took her mind back to the mission in Zambia where she had served as a medical missionary, remembering Janet as a baby at that mission. The baby had thrived, matured, and in that Spring of 1994 was seeking additional training before returning to serve the Lord at a school for missionaries' children in Zambia.

The following year, however, only two full-time and one part-time students enrolled for the courses, although they were themselves on a time budget of just one month!

After much prayer and discussion at the end of 1995, the Council decided with great reluctance to discontinue advertising training at Hahnemann House and *'to venture to widen its ministry as the Lord leads'*.

But it was not the conclusion of the MSM after all! Early in the next year the following Press Release was published:

Press Release - May 1996: Responding to Changing Circumstances Medical Service Ministries offers Christian workers a new resource.

> Established in 1903 for the training of persons proposing to serve as missionaries abroad, MSM now offers guidance for those seeking qualifications and skills in the area of personal health care and community care.

For Christian workers and accredited missionaries seeking such training, guidance is available, appropriate for their circumstances and requirements. In appropriate cases, MSM offers grants to those who undertake approved training courses.

After successfully training more than fifteen hundred personnel from many different backgrounds with a wide range of professional skills, MSM now concentrates on assisting those whose interests range from first-aid through to tropical diseases.

Guidance in basic health training represents a valuable resource for Christian workers seeking to respond to Christ's commission to 'preach and heal'.

All enquiries should be addressed to:
The Candidate Secretary, Medical Service Missionaries
P.O.Box 35, Hailsham, East Sussex, BN27 3XW
Tel/Fax 01323 849047

**Friends are invited to write for supplies of the MSM brochure
detailing this new development.**

Vacating No.2 for the Last Time
Throughout the years of the twentieth century the Missionary School of Medicine had for much of that time occupied all the rooms of No.2 Powis Place, but in more recent years, as the number of students declined, the School had relinquished most of them to the Faculty of Homoeopathy. However, its three rooms *at the top of the house* all contained furniture and equipment which now needed to be sold or distributed to other missions or to churches. Initially, this seemed a mammoth task. Not only was the furniture antique and therefore very heavy, but everything was on the third floor *of a house with a winding stairway.*

As the Warden listed everything, and prayed about it all, little by little these problems began to be solved. Faith can remove mountains, therefore why not the MSM furniture?

For a number of years it had been desired to remove the piano but various removal firms had refused. With regard to the antique furniture, it was decided to call upon Sotheby's for their expert advice, which was duly given. Four items were to go under the hammer for auction; a roll-top desk, a carved bookcase, a French clock and the piano. Two men arrived one morning to carry the items away. It took them forty minutes to take the piano down the stairway. The Secretary's heart was in her mouth most of the time for fear of any damage to the men, one of whom already had a bad back. Once it was on the lorry, Jean was able to refresh them with a cup of tea. They could have done with a shower!

All the items were duly sold and the MSM funds boosted. *(At the end, the proceeds of the various sales exceeded the cost of vacating the premises and removing a minimal amount to Hailsham.)* By this time, the Secretary had one empty office apart from a table and various odds and ends.

A number of missions were contacted to offer them medical equipment and the Secretary received a greater response than she could manage. Desks, chairs, video, TV and the OHP were offered to local, known churches. All were snapped up and it was quite amazing to see how the Lord undertook in all this. There never was any doubt in anyone's mind but that they were doing the right thing. It all went so smoothly.

While emptying the cupboards on the landing where most of the School's literature was stored, a portrait of Hudson Taylor, the founder of the China Inland Mission, was discovered. Mrs Hayward-Lynch contacted the historian for that Mission to see if they would like it, and when they replied in the affirmative it was promptly dispatched. At the same time another portrait, this time of Dr David Livingstone, was found together with the plaster cast of his wounded forearm, previously referred to. These valued items were forwarded to the Livingstone Museum in Glasgow.

A certain amount of equipment was needed to set up the Candidate Secretary's office in Hailsham, East Sussex and a number of friends from her home church helped in the transportation of these. *There remained just one item, the photocopier - and one problem -* ***those stairs at No.2!***

One evening, Mrs Jean Hayward-Lynch and two friends attempted to carry the photocopier down the winding stairway, only to sustain one strained back, one snapped sternum and torn rib muscles before reaching the second floor! The copier went no further for six weeks, while the Secretary recovered from her injuries and was then able to call in a skilled removal firm to complete the task.

The library of devotional and missionary books was given to the Redcliffe Missionary Training College. Homoeopathic books, mainly good Materia Medica, along with a much cherished portrait of Samuel Hahnemann which had hung in the office for many years, were donated to the Hahnemann Museum.

With the help of Mavis Knowles all the School's obsolete records were packed into two large wooden chests. They comprised student and examination registers, reports, memoirs of Miss Bargh and Miss Bottom and a number of other historical items. These were deposited with the Archivist at the School for Oriental and African Studies in London.

Last, but not least, that which remained had to come under the heading of scrap - the Gestetner duplicator and old-style steel stands, at one time used to hold teaching equipment. As it was thought scrap metal was valuable a London based firm of scrap-metal dealers was called in. How wrong can one be. The School was charged sixty pounds to have it all removed.

So it was that on 19th June 1996, Mrs Hayward-Lynch handed over the keys of Hahnemann House, No.2 Powis Place, for the last time and the lease was duly surrendered.

It was indeed the conclusion of the 'Missionary School of Medicine'.
What a wonderful story, spanning 93 years! Indeed, 'TO GOD BE THE
GLORY! GREAT THINGS HE HAS DONE!'
*But it was also a NEW BEGINNING for Medical Service Ministries.
And the famous acronym that unites the PAST with the FUTURE is
MSM.*

So our story continues.

A Case of MetaMorphoSe
The discerning eye will notice familiar letters (albeit in a different
sequence) in this word indicating a 'Change of Form'. The May 1996
press release already quoted, outlined the continuation of this story
through the radical changes which MSM then passed. It moved from
being essentially a Lay-Missionary-Medical-Teaching-School to a
Grant-making Advisory Trust for prospective mission partners in a
changing world. In this new mode MSM continues to help prospective
and active Christian workers. It is the conviction of the Trustees (the
members of Council) that it will continue to receive the support of
many friends, and not least of course, that the Lord of the Harvest will
be pleased to bless and prosper the work and resources he has entrusted
to them.

On surrendering the Lease of the top floor at Hahnemann House MSM
operated through the voluntary efforts of the Trustees - no premises -
no staff. It was a great help to the Trust in its new role to have the
continued assistance of Mrs Jean Hayward-Lynch, the former Head of
Studies and Secretary, who immediately following her retirement from
those duties agreed to act as the Candidate Secretary. Her wide
experience over many years enabled her to undertake this sensitive task
with great understanding and care and she was warmly welcomed to
join the Council as an additional Trustee. The work of the Lord
continued, giving encouragement and assisting the training of those he
calls to go forth into all the world to 'preach and heal'.

Six years after surrendering that Lease, with MSM becoming more
widely known, it became clear to the trustees that their work needed to
be consolidated in one place and pushed forward with more vigour and
single mindedness than the two most active (on behalf of MSM) of
their number, being septagenarians, were likely to achieve.   Thus at
the commencement of the Centenary year its office moved to Ware,

with the candidate bureau and other administrative functions being undertaken by Mrs Glennis A. Dowling, an experienced and committed Christian worker.

How Medical Service Ministries Functions
From the MSM Resource Bureau missionary candidates and others seeking the better to equip themselves for the Lord's service, in candidates' home countries and elsewhere, can obtain addresses and contact names for a range of courses on offer in the UK. In time a similar list of suitable courses on offer in other sending countries will be compiled. MSM also has a booklist, of interest to any desirous of undertaking private study. This includes titles which will sometimes be helpful for reference when at work overseas without clinic, doctor or hospital nearby.

When applying for training grants, candidates must be able to subscribe to the published statement of faith which appears on page 164 and be sponsored by a Christian mission or community, prior to acceptance by MSM for an approved course.

Finance
The Trustees operate a policy of openness in all matters, seeking first and foremost to walk in paths opened up by our heavenly Father for the advancement of the Kingdom of Christ in every area of life. Consequently, they have not felt it necessary or wise to make public appeal for funds, because they are convinced that those whom the Lord directs will know his will in their personal stewardship of this world's goods, acknowledging that they and all they possess are his own. The trustees, nevertheless, seek to extend public awareness of the world-wide needs and opportunities which remain to be addressed.

Down through the years, freewill gifts and legacies were received for the maintenance of the School and to ameliorate student fees through the Bursary Fund. Subsequently, the Scholarship Fund was launched, on the School's 90th anniversary, with the theme of 'thanksgiving', for the sole purpose of awarding grants for approved training undertaken by approved candidates. Unless otherwise directed, the Trustees will credit to the Scholarship Fund all gifts of £1,000 or more to directly benefit those able, under the terms of its Constitution, to receive MSM training grants.

An *approved* course is one which offers additional training, for missionaries and other Christian workers called to serve, in the area of personal, and/or child, and/or community health care. In the past MSM courses did not advance the professional training of Christians, of any nationality, other than by assisting where additional qualifications were necessary to enable candidates to undertake duties and further the gospel through evangelical Christian organisations or communities. Proof of 'call' and evidence of sponsorship continue to be required. MSM interprets *community* to include local companies of believers covenanting together to seek the mind of Christ and to communicate the love of God in the power of the Holy Spirit.

A Change of President

The Council saw many changes during the five years up to 1998 which followed the School's 90th anniversary. During all that rather traumatic time it was so ably and spiritually guided by its President, the Revd T. Omri Jenkins. At the end of that period, he wrote:

> *My years are climbing and what may be left for me I hope to use to preach as opportunities occur. My hope and prayer are that MSM's many friends will continue to support and pray for its work in the coming days and that God will be glorified in and through all its endeavours.*

So it was, with much thanksgiving, that the Trustees were led to appoint Mr Edwin Orton, a previous student of the MSM, to the office of President to continue the task which the Revd T.Omri Jenkins relinquished after five years of devoted service. After successful church planting work in Essex, Mr Orton became a founder member of the Birmingham City Mission, which began in 1966, and he is involved in similar City Mission work overseas. His vision and enthusiasm for the new role being undertaken by the Medical Service Ministries augurs well for its anticipated future ministry and development. This is best expressed in the following,

Mission Statement

> *To encourage full-time Christian workers in the UK and elsewhere to prepare for Personal and Community Healthcare work in the developing world, in association with Christian organisations, and to witness to their faith in obedience to Christ's command to preach and heal. Funding is available for approved healthcare candidates.*

Authorised Grants to date
From the launch of the Scholarship Fund in 1993 to the end of September 2002 more than £50,000 has been authorised for healthcare and related professional training for a variety of applicants. Grants are small or large depending upon the type and duration of the studies involved and the circumstances of the applicants. All are carefully assessed by the Trustees after much prayer and careful thought. Appendix E provides details.

This History of the MSM closes with a fine testimony from one of these successful applicants. **Sharon Liu** is a mature Christian nurse, who came to Liverpool in 1999, from China to achieve an ambitious goal. Now she is able to rejoice that in God's wonderful strength, she has been able to gain a Master's degree in Community Health which has equipped her to train others.

'Like Eating an Elephant!'
Sharing the burden of projects aimed at improved community health in a remote mountainous region, Sharon undertook the journey to the UK relying upon God alone to provide all the resources necessary. Along with others MSM was pleased to be instrumental, but only the Lord was able to direct her path, empower her intellect and will to study in a relatively unknown tongue and, all the while, encourage her through contacts with his Spirit-filled people. Sharon readily acknowledges that the unstinting kindness of ex-missionaries, many different landladies, an elderly couple gifted with an inspiring Bible ministry, even the unspoken ministry of springtime and harvest, together with the plan of the Lord to keep her in Liverpool while writing her dissertation, all contributed to her success.

Tenacity and devotion to the Lord's calling is evident. She likened writing her dissertation to eating an elephant, whose tail was tasty but too long. She asks our prayers for her family, with whom she spent some months before resuming work, for her sending church and for *'The Lord's will and not human planning.'*

The needs are tremendous, but Sharon is now better equipped to address them. She does not work alone. Team members have benefited from this new found knowledge. As a Registered Nurse she has helped in the local hospital and in various rural health projects, including

142

youth work and animal welfare. Those who have first-hand knowledge of her industry testify that she has not spared herself to visit people in need. Recently she wrote,

> Once I had a small room I was able to put my bed, which was a child's mattress, on the floor. It was cosy and comfortable. I realised that I do not take up a lot of space when I lie down. Yes, this reminds me to ask, 'How much space a person needs in their life?' Recently, the message of Matthew 11:28 has spoken to me - being gentle and humble in heart, we find rest for our soul and the yoke is lighter. Working alongside Jesus, His yoke is easy and His burden is light - Jesus, Light of the world.

A new beginning marks the end of this book and all that has been recounted in these pages has been but a preparation for it. We may well ponder what will be revealed of this story in another hundred years. Perhaps the reader will have some influence upon it, by taking advantage of MSM's desire to be of assistance to those who seek to embody Christ in a challenging situation overseas, or by gifting funds to make this possible for others.

'Maranatha!'

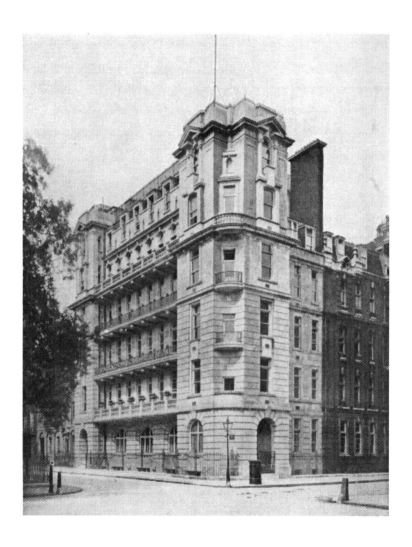

The Royal London Homoeopathic Hospital
The Original Home of the School

Appendix A

Much more than a friend

The Royal London Homoeopathic Hospital

Several times in the course of this History mention has been made of the ready access which students were afforded to the Royal London Homoeopathic Hospital. A briefly outline of some of the significant changes which took place during the 100 years described in this book may be of interest to readers.

The Hospital began in 1849 with some thirty-five or forty beds in Golden Square, London, but it soon outgrew its borders and was transferred to Great Ormond Street, Bloomsbury, where it occupied one of the fine old private houses in that once fashionable street. It was the house occupied by Zachary Macaulay, the philanthropist, and father of Lord Macaulay, the historian and politician. It was here that William Wilberforce and his colleagues of the anti-slavery struggle had their headquarters. The marble hall and staircase formed an imposing entrance to the little hospital.

In 1859 the hospital acquired three adjacent houses, and two extensions brought it into the adjoining Queen's Square, with a total of 170 beds. Increase in efficiency kept pace with increase in size. Again in 1893, a more up-to-date building was necessary and the Board of Management were able, by the magnanimous gifts of many benefactors, to open a newly-built hospital on the same site, free of debt, containing the latest scientific and hospital equipment. It was into this building that the Missionary School of Medicine was welcomed when it was founded in 1903. Then in 1911, a new wing was added to the hospital, named the Sir Henry Tyler extension, which not only gave a handsome frontage in Queen's Square but provided additional wards and Administrative accommodation.

At this time the Hospital had three operating theatres. The outpatients' department had a series of general and special consulting rooms - well known to MSM students - an up-to-date Xray department, a mechanotherapy clinic, surgical dressings room, almoner's office, dispensary and waiting hall. The ground floor had one ward (male medical), the pathological laboratory and lecture room, porters' office, casualty rooms, waiting room, administration offices, two electric lifts, staff room and board room. In the last named handsome and spacious room, MSM students sat with postgraduate doctors for certain lectures. The remaining floors were devoted chiefly to wards, medical and surgical. Further extensions were carried out in 1923-33 under the direction of Prof. Beresford Pite enabling the hospital to have 200 beds, and giving it the reputation of being one of the most modern hospitals in London.

In 1980, due to financial cutbacks, the Hospital had to close its main operating theatre and a number of surgical wards, but the fortunes of the hospital improved a few years later and it was able to greatly improve its outpatient facilities with seven new modern clinics, a physiotherapy department and a pharmacy.

In 1993 it became an independent autonomous trust within the NHS which allowed many changes and improvements to be undertaken. These included the creation of an academic department with directors of research and education, extended services and the establishment of the first NHS musculoskeletal department.

In 1999 the Hospital joined the Parkside Health NHS Community Trust operating in central and west London. Due to Central Government administrative policy this Trust is no longer in existence.

In April 2002 the Hospital merged with University College London Hospital Group to share accommodation with the Royal Orthopaedic Hospital. It is intended that the Royal London Homoeopathic Hospital's complementary therapies, including homoeopathy, will continue into the 21st Century and that it will be numbered among the largest medical, educational and research centres in Europe. The plan is that this £18.5 million redevelopment should be completed in 2004.

Appendix B

Officials and Staff for the 30th Session of the School, 1933-1934

President The Revd J. Stuart Holden MA, DD,

Vice-Presidents
J. Benson Bear FRCS,
Miss Blomfield
E. Clifton Brown JP.
R.H.Caird JP.
The Countess of Clanwilliam
Sir Henry Davenport JP.
Revd C.E. Hurlburt
Revd J.D. Jones CH,MA,DD,
Sir Robert Perks Bt.
Professor Beresford Pite
MA,FRIBA,
W.H.Poate
Miss A.W. Richardson BA,
The Countess Roberts
F. Howard Taylor MD, FRCS,
James W. Thirtle LLD, DD,
Sir G. Wyatt Truscott Bt.☐

General Council
H.B. Bilbrough
Mrs Boake
Clarence H.M. Foster MA,
Revd H.S. Gamman
Miss K. Goodin (Secretary)
Montague Goodman
Ernest Grimwood
Miss Agnes Keep
A. Stuart McNairn FRGS,
F.W. Miller
Frank Piper
Miss Edna Wills
F.Marcus Wood☐

Executive Committee
D.M. Borland MB,
George Burford MB, CM,
A.T. Cunningham MB, ChB,
V.T. Ellwood MA, MD,
Montague Goodman Esq.
Vincent Green MD,
C. Granville Hey MB, CM,
A. Stuart McNairn FRGS,
Edwin A. Neatby MD, (Dean)
T. Pearson MRCS, DOMS Lond.
J.C. Powell MRCS,
Margaret L .Tyler MD,
Sir John Weir KCVO, MB, (Chairman)

Teaching Staff

Dorothy Anderson MRCS, LRCP,
Horace W. Applin MB,
Helena F. Banks MB, ChB,
Geraldine Barry MS Lond. FRCS,
J.W. Bell LRCP, LRCSI,
Alva Benjamin MB, ChM,
Margery Blackie MD, BS Lond.
D.M. Borland MB, ChB,
Cecil Burnham FRCS Edin.
A.T. Cunningham MB, ChB,
A.H. Margaret Denton MB, BS,
James Eadie FRCS,
V.T. Ellwood MA, MD Oxon.
D.S. Gordon MB, BCh, BAO
Belfast,
Martha Griffith BSc, MB,
Edith M. Hall MD Lond. BS,
Tatiana Hardy MBC,
C. Granville Hey MB, CM,
H.W. Hill LDSRCS,
D. Morgan Hughes FRCS,

J.D. Kenyon MB, BCh,
D.A. McCombie MB,
W.R. McCrae MB, ChB,
A.D.C. MacGowan MB, ChB,
J. C. MacKillop MB, ChB Glas.
W.B.D. Miller MB, ChB,
Agnes Moncrief MB, ChB Glas.
T. Miller Neatby MA, MD Cantab.
T. Pearson MRCS, LRCP, DOMS,
P.G.Quinton MD Lond.
J.M. Rishworth MB, BCh,
Maurice Robinson MB, BCh,
W.W. Rorke MB, ChB,
A.R. Stacey LDSRCS,
W. Lees Templeton MD, ChB,
Margaret L. Tyler MD,
John Weir KCVO, MB, ChB,
C.E. Wheeler MD, BSc Lond.
H. Fergie Woods MD,

Appendix C

A Christian Doctor Looks at Homoeopathy

By Dr. Anita E. Davies, MB, BS, MRCP, DRCOG, FFHom.
First printed 'IN THE SERVICE OF MEDICINE' the Journal of The Christian Medical Fellowship Vol. 32:3 No.127 July 1986.

Dr. Davies is a MSM Council Member.

As a Christian and a doctor the author has common ground with the majority who will read this article. As a physician using homoeopathy I am in the minority. There are under 700 members and associates of the Faculty of Homoeopathy - the body set up by Act of Parliament in 1950 when the National Health Service came into being. The Faculty holds examinations for Membership and Fellowship, sets professional standards, and runs post graduate educational courses. An association of doctors has existed since the 1830s when a Dr. Hervey Quinn introduced Homoeopathy into England. He founded the first Homoeopathic Hospital in London in 1850, about the same time as the British Medical Association was formed. There has always been much professional jealousy and opposition, but in spite of this the teaching and practice of homoeopathic medicine by medical graduates has continued uninterrupted to the present day.

There were soon hospitals in Bristol, Glasgow, Liverpool and Tunbridge Wells, all of which are flourishing today and part of the National Health Service. Others, such as the Birmingham Homoeopathic Hospital, have disappeared, but at Selly Oak Hospital Post Graduate Centre there is an active branch of the Faculty of Homoeopathy teaching the principles and practice of homoeopathic medicine to an ever growing number of Midland doctors.

Christian Doubt

Recently in some Christian circles doubts have been expressed about Homoeopathy, linking it with occult medical practice such as Yoga and Transcendental Meditation. This has arisen out of consideration of its origins and certain associations which have attached themselves to homoeopathic practice during its long history. Richard Macaulay discusses this in *Christian Women* (pp 18-21 October 1985) quoting

Hahnemann and citing a 'vital force' in human beings which becomes 'deranged' in illness and is restored to balance by a 'spiritual force' said to be released during the preparation of the homoeopathic remedy. Another article condemns Hahnemann for 'his dedication to Freemasonry and his identification with eastern religions' (from *Message for our Times Teaching Articles* No.5).

The use of the pendulum in diagnosis and in choice of treatment is by some considered occult as is the influence of Rudolf Steiner and the Anthroposophical Movement on the preparation of some medicines used in homoeopathy[1]. However homoeopathy should not be mis-judged because of the people who practise it nor be mis-interpreted because of a cultural link with an eighteenth century philosophical style, or because of the religious beliefs - or lack of them - of its founder. After all, many advances in science and medicine have been made by non-Christians and they are not therefore invalid. Common grace allows us all to benefit from advancing knowledge.

It is nevertheless historically true that religious reform and awakening to the Christian Gospel precedes scientific revelation, and was particularly evident at the Reformation which preceded discoveries of William Hervey and others from which modern medicine takes its roots. There are besides a large number of active Christians who personally make use of homoeopathy and find it an aid to recovery from ill health.

What is homoeopathic medicine?

There are two main principles which underlie the use of medicine in homoeopathy:

1 The Similia Principle -
    i.e. a substance which can cause a symptom complex in a healthy
        person can be used to treat a similar complex of symptoms in a
        sick person.

2 The Dose -
    the quantity of medicine should be the smallest possible to effect a
        cure and should not be repeated as long as improvement lasts.

Plants and other natural products of animal or mineral origin have been the basis of all primitive medicines since man was created and was subject to injury and pain. Ancient Egyptian, Chinese, Hindu and Greek manuscripts describe the traditional use of such substances.

Hippocrates wrote in about 460BC of the use of plants which produce toxic symptoms in some species of animals being used to cure the same syndrome in man. The Bible speaks of healing plants 'Their fruit will serve for food and their leaves for healing'[2].

Dr. Samuel Hahnemann (1775-1843) was a linguist, a chemist and a doctor. In his translation work he collected a number of references to healing by 'similars' and fully acknowledged that he was not the first to discover this. He investigated the action of medical substances used in his day by taking small doses himself and giving the same to members of his family and friends, some of whom were doctors. A systematic record of the symptoms produced was kept in a formal 'schema' following the anatomy of the body. When a sick person presented with a similar set of symptoms, the medicine was given and repeatedly the sick person was seen to recover.

Altogether Hahnemann spent about ten years recording these results before publishing his discovery in a leading medical journal of his day[3]. Because in some instances the patient became worse before he got better the dose was reduced. With poisonous substances- like white arsenic (which was recognized as an adulterant of wine in his day)- it was necessary to reduce the dose considerably. Hahnemann found that by diluting the substance in an alcohol- water solution by serial steps of 1 in 10 or 1 in 100, the effect of the medicine was enhanced. Being a chemist he naturally shook the bottle between dilutions to ensure thorough mixing. He called these 'potencies' and used medicines in dilutions ranging from 10^{-12} to 10^{-60}.

Hahnemann's initial work was based entirely on observation and experiment and he disclaimed speculation. Later when he left the stimulating environment of Leipzig University he introduced his own philosophy into homoeopathic medicine to explain how it might work. He was greatly influenced by the Swedenborgian philosophy as was his chief follower James Tyler Kent who practised medicine in the United States. Their writings reflect the nineteenth-century language and intellectual climate. It is not surprising that terms such as 'vital force' should be used to explain both the development of symptoms (when the person's equilibrium was deranged) and their treatment by the potentized medicine which was assumed to act by restoring the 'vital force' to normal. Surely what Hahnemann was referring to was the homoeostatic mechanism which we now know something about and which is constantly at work maintaining and promoting health.

The Organon

In his treatise *The Organon* Hahnemann describes what a physician should be and do, how to take a history and prescribe a homoeopathic medicine, and how to remove '*obstacles to cure*' both by means of hygiene and an orderly way of living and by dealing with the cause of chronic disease. He postulated a chronic 'miasm' (again a nineteenth-century term meaning a 'taint') bringing about chronic illness in certain constitutions. He identified syphilis and gonorrhonea as two and scabies as a third.

He experimented with a further group of medicines for chronic disease to deal with these miasms. This idea of hereditary predisposition together with an infective element precipitating a chronic illness was quite novel when first postulated, but has recently been corroborated in diseases such as chronic wart infections, where an immune deficiency prevents viral warts being thrown off quickly[4]. This syndrome matches Hahnemann's gonorrhoea type illness - Sycosis as he called it.

Dr. Margaret Blackie, who was one of the most brilliant homoeopathic physicians of the 20th Century, wrote:

> Homoeopathy has not changed at all since Hahnemann founded it, and since it has not been affected by all the modern knowledge it is thought to be obsolete. Medicine, on the other hand, is advancing dramatically every year. But as I wander between Hahnemann's *Organon* and modern medical journals I conclude that homoeopathy started in advance and that orthodox medical knowledge has not yet caught it up.
> (From *Classical Homoeopathy* edited by Dr. Charles Elliot and Dr. Frank Johnson, p37, published by Beaconsfield 1986).

Research

Present day research is particularly looking at the following questions:

1 How is it that medicines, diluted well below any possibility of a molecule of the original substance being present, have any healing effect?

2 Does a homoeopathic medicine have any more effect than a placebo? If it does, how does it work?

The first question was tackled using a model of hay fever. Dr. David Reilly has conducted two trials both with positive results, showing that a homoeopathic preparation of Mixed Pollens in a 30c 10^{-60} dilution given to patients suffering from hay fever relieves symptoms more favourably than a placebo[5].

The second question has been tackled by Dr. K.R.Keysell using a standard analgesic laboratory test comparing the effect of Hypericum and Arnica with Morphine. The results showed that Hypericum 30c relieved pain significantly better than placebo and moreover the effect could be eliminated by giving Naloxone[6]. This implicates opioid systems in the body and suggests a possible mode of action for homoeopathy. This excites the imagination and deserves further investigation.

In this way research is beginning to confirm the clinical impression gained by many physicians that a homoeopathic medicine stimulates the healing response more effectively than does a placebo. Nevertheless it is also true that the doctor-patient encounter is in itself a stimulus to recovery. All doctors have the possibility of using their consultations for teaching, when personal life styles and environmental factors responsible for much ill health can be discussed and many eliminated. The homoeopathic doctor is also interested in the patient's perception of his illness in general and the mental charcteristics which reflect his constitutional make up, as well as in the particular physical manifestations from which a clinical diagnosis is made. We each have a personal finger print and genetic make up which is unique. It is the aim of the homoeopathic doctor to identify the personal profile of the patient and make a prescription which covers the 'totality of symptoms' - both the pathology and the personality.

An Example

We can look at white arsenic (the homoeopathic Arsenicum Album) which causes diarrhoea and vomiting in acute poisonous doses, but in chronic poisoning develops a sickness well characterised in the victims in J.O.Kesselring's *Arsenic and Old Lace*. This medicine was used effectively in very dilute dosage during the second world war for trench diarrhoea, and many families have it in their medicine chests in a homoeopathic preparation for acute food poisoning. However it can also be used in chronic illness, be it a chest complaint like asthma or bronchitis, or a digestive problem like duodenal ulcer or colitis, or a mental illness such as anxiety depression.

For arsenic to be effective as a remedy, the patient must fulfil certain characteristics. The General Symptoms include reaction to temperature: the patient is chilly and hates the cold, he has certain aversions and desires for food, he enjoys eating fat, he has specific personality traits, such as being restless and fastidious. Mentally he is a very anxious person, full of fears. In such a patient a few doses of high potency Arsenicum Album 10^{-60} or higher will improve his general health and well being and relapses in his chronic illness will be less frequent.

A psycho-somatic approach

Hahnemann recognised the importance of psychological symptoms in illness and was one of the pioneers of the humane treatment of mentally ill patients. Homoeopathy was the first system of medicine to develop a psycho-somatic approach to illness, the medicines prescribed having been chosen taking into account all the information available. Objective validation of this approach has been demonstrated by Galen Ives, a clinical psychologist, in respect of half-a-dozen homoeopathic medicines (out of some 200 in common use) and it is at present being investigated further in a University Psychology Department[7].

For what, by whom?

So what sort of patients do we see and what sort of doctors practise homoeopathy? An ever increasing number of young medical graduates are coming to learn the principles at the Faculty's Courses in London, Bristol and Glasgow. In a recent survey of General Practitioner Trainees[8] over 50% expressed an interest in learning one of the complementary therapies. A report on a National Survey of Homoeopathic practice in the United Kingdom conducted in 1982[9] showed the wide variety of medical conditions treated. When modern therapy was effective, as in bacterial infections and hypertension, conventional treatment was used, but in self limiting illnesses and in allergies and in chronic non-responding conditions, homoeopathic medicine was more likely to be prescribed. Undergraduate medical students have chosen homoeopathy as their special study and come from as faraway as New Zealand. During a morning consultation with one such student the author saw three children with eczema, two with upper respiratory infections; adults with anxiety depression, arthritis, proctitis, obesity and dementia. A dozen different homoeopathic medicines were prescribed, and special investigations undertaken in one patient with panic attacks to confirm the clinical diagnosis of chronic hypocarbia, a diagnosis which is often overlooked. When a patient fails to respond to the indicated medicine there is often some physical or psychological disorder which in traditional homoeopathy is called 'an obstacle to cure.'

Supplying the deficiency (e.g. B12), remedying the overbreathing or correcting the displaced vertebra, or giving psychotherapy, anti depressant or anti psychotic medicine is essential before the patient recovers. The part that the homoeopathic medicine plays in such patients has not been objectively assessed, but it can replace the use of the addictive benzodiazepans. The individualisation of each patient enables a medicine to be prescribed which covers all aspects of his complaint in the one prescription. This is well illustrated in the multiple symptomatology of the hyperventilation syndrome[10].

In conclusion

One can see that homoeopathy is a form of complementary medicine which utilises all one's medical skills yet provides a simple and non-toxic form of treatment for many self-limiting illnesses, the toxicity of poisons having been removed through the process of serial dilution and succession which is used in manufacturing the medicine. It offers relief when orthodox medicine often has to say 'there is little more we can do.'

In some of these patients the homoeopathic concept of chronic disease opens up therapeutic possibilities which have not yet been fully developed. In chronic disease in particular, the patient and doctor share the responsibilities of restoring health, for only as the patient reveals all his symptoms and feelings can the doctor choose from a large repertoire of medicines - which have their own 'drug pictures' - that one which matches the indiviudal patient most closely.

As in all medicine, the doctor may have to revise his clinical diagnosis in the light of the patient's response to treatment, and in so doing exercises that truly Christian virtue of humility.

'Let this mind be in you which was also in Christ Jesus'[11].

References

[1] Isaiah 8:19

[2] Ezekiel 47:12

[3] The Essay on a New Principle for Ascertaining the Curative Powers of Drugs and Some Examinations of the Previous Principles; *Hufeland's Journal* Vol.2 pieces 3 and 4, pp 391-439, 465-561, 1796; Listed in *Samuel Hahnemann His Life and Works, Vol 2 by Richard Hael.*

[4] Throwing off Warts, editorial *British Medical Journal, August 19th, 1978,* p521.

[5] Potent Placebo or Potency, David Taylor Reilly et al, *British Homoeopathic Journal*, Vol.74 No.2, pp65-75, April 1985.

[6] An Investigation into the Analgesic Activity of two Homoeopathic Preparations, Arnica and Hypericum, G R Keysall et al *Communications* No.11 (Journal of the Midlands (now British) Homoeopathy Research Group) BHRG, pp32-48.

[7] An Empirical Validation of the Homoeopathic Theory of Type, Galen Ives, *Proceedings of the 35th Congress of the Liga Medicorum Homoeopathica Internationalis,* 1982, pp 148-161.

[8] Young Doctors Views of Alternative Medicines, David Taylor Reilly, *British Medical Journal,* 1983, Vol.287, pp337-339.

[9] Homoeopathic Practice in the UK, Philip Nicholls *Communications* No.13, (Journal of the BHRG).

[10] Homoeopathic Medicine in the treatment of chronic hypocapnoea, Anita Davies, *British Homoeopathic Journal,* Vol LXVII, No.1, Jan 1978.

[11] Philippians 2:5

Appendix D

Science Offers a Solution to Homoeopathy

By Robert Uhlig, Technology Correspondent
Quoted with permission from 'The Daily Telegraph' 8-11-2001

A chance discovery that has amazed chemists might provide scientific evidence to prove that homoeopathy is not suspect after all.

Homoeopaths repeatedly dilute remedies, believing that the higher the dilution the more potent it becomes, until at infinite dilution the solution is more potent than the original active ingredient.

Scientists have always disclaimed this argument, partly because common sense dictates that the solution is so diluted that none of the active ingredient remains.

Now a team of scientists based in South Korea has inadvertently discovered that dissolved molecules cluster together as the solution is diluted. When the solution is diluted further, the clusters clump together to form even larger clusters.

Kurt Geckeler, a chemist, and his colleague, Shashadhar Samal, stumbled on the effect while investigating ullerenes, huge carbon molecules, at the Kwangju Institute of Science and Technology.

The finding, double-checked and confirmed with electron microscopy, goes against conventional wisdom and years of teaching that molecules disperse farther apart the more the solution is diluted.

The *New Scientist* reported: 'The finding may provide a mechanism for how some homoeopathic medicines work, something that has defied scientific explanation till now.'

Appendix E

Statement of Authorised Grants

Grantee	Nationality	Sponsor

Grantee	Nationality	Sponsor
Satisfied MSM admissions criterea	British	AIM
From Northumbria Bible College	Korean	Home church
Street children ministry, Brazil	British	UFM
Physician half time with OM	British	OM
Professional for Romanian charity	Romanian	MSM
Physician	British	OM
Christian hospital worker	Zambian	Mambilima
From Word of Life Mission Inst.	Brazilian	MEIB
Christian Nurse	Taiwanese	InterHealth
Nurse with links to West Africa	British	TEAR Fund
Africa Inland Church project	British	AIM
Nurse in rural health programme	Ghanian	Home church
From working in Kosovo	British	YWAM
Physician from Mission Hosp.	Nigerian	Qua Iboe
Physicians voluntarily with PRIME	British	Romanian CMF
Nurse having studied at MSM	British	Mildmay Uganda
Nurse following studies at YWAM	British	Mercy Ships
From Asian relief programmes	British	Various
Physicians voluntarily with PRIME	British	Albanian CMA
From voluntary work in Benin	British	Mercy Ships

Grants subsequently authorised

Grantee	Nationality	Sponsor
Nurse Midwife from Dev. studies	Tanzanian	Home church
From Medical studies, Bristol	British	Crosslinks
Dr. originally with AEF	British	SIM
Dr. with Africa Inland Church	British	AIM
Physicians volunteering their services	British	PRIME
Hospital worker from Livingstonia	Malawian	EMMS
Nurse developing community training	Liberian	Lifeline
Dr. with Servants to Asia's Urban Poor	NZ	Home church
Student nurse for tribal work	Argentina	Iglesia Anglicana
Student nurse for tribal work	Argentina	Iglesia Anglicana
Occupational therapist	British	MECCO
Physician serving in Asia	British	OMF

Grant   Details of Course

£1,570	Autumn 1995 at MSM
£1,566	Advance Health & Social Care - Gateshead
£ 370	Tropical Medicine for Nurses - Liverpool
£1,067	Diploma in Travel Medicine - Glasgow
£ 750	Homoeopathy - Royal London Homoeopathic Hosp.
£1,258	MSc. in Travel Medicine - Glasgow
£ 832	Dispensing Asst. - Evelyn Hone, Lusaka
£2,460	Nurse Technician - Omega Professional - Belem, Pará
£6,150	MSc. Community Health - Liverpool
£3,000	Disaster Relief Nursing - University of Coleraine, 3 yrs
£2,000	Kenyan HIV/AIDS Secondary Sch. Teachers for peers
£ 260	CMF course for nurses and midwives
£ 195	Tropical Medicine - Liverpool.
£1,460	Dip.s Trop. Med. & International Health - Dublin
£ 500	Travel expenses to doctors' conference and courses
£ 700	Palliative care Manchester University
£1,224	Univ.London Child to Child Trust health promotion
£2,500	MSc. International Health - Queen Margaret Univ.Col.
£ 500	Travel expenses to doctors' conference and courses
£ 750	Dip.Trop.Med. - London Sch.Hygiene & Tropical Med.

£2,737	MA. Primary Health Care - Royal Col.Surgeons, Dublin
£ 450	Trop.Med. prior to clinic project in Tanzania
£ 500	Refresher studies at CMDA Conference in Kenya
£ 500	XIV International AIDS Conf. assisting Kenyan Church
£2.565	International medical education - Albania, Romania & Hungary
£3,000	MA. in Public Health in South Africa
£ 700	CMF refresher course
£2,500	MA. in Public Health and child health research and development
US$6,000	Enfermera Profesional
US$6,000	Enfermera Profesional
£1,300	Training to work with Children with Cerebral Palsy
£ 925	Diploma in Tropical Medicine & Hygiene

Appendix F

The Lord's Provision

Six year aggregates
(sum of annual surpluses and deficits)

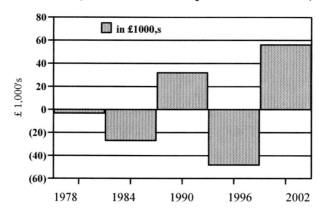

The above diagram illustrates the fluctuations in annual accounts for the thirty years up to 30 September 2002.   To show the trend more clearly the period is divided into five six-year periods, with the final period covering the six years since MSM training in London ceased. The figures in brackets relate to the three periods when annual deficits exceeded annual surpluses. Had the school continued beyond 1996 it is estimated that deficits would have continued at the rate of £10,000 per annum. Prior to these thirty years the fluctuations were insignificant.

During the years up to 1990 the Lord graciously endowed the school through the generosity of supporters who had bequeathed funds, the total of which exceeded operating deficits. Not one of the subsequent six years showed a surplus. During the final six years MSM's annual accounts reflected the award of training grants totalling £48,000.

The growth and separation of funds, representing the assets of MSM, is shown below.

MSM ASSETS

□ Endowment Fund
□ Investment Fund
□ General Fund with related School Funds
□ General Investment Reserve
▨ Scholarship Funds - cash plus investments

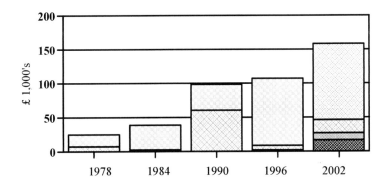

0The diagram above depicts the years featured on the previous page. Unlike the previous diagram, what is shown is the relative growth in funds, comparing year with year. The situation during intervening years is not shown. Due to inflation over the twenty-four years between 1978 and 2002 this growth is illusory.

However, the appearance of Scholarship Funds following the 90th Anniversary Thanksgiving Appeal should be noted:
        1996 - £1,899   *2002* - £16,621
illustrated above at the bottom of the two last columns, but too small to be visible in the 1996 column.

Investments grew; as the result of legacies and favourable stock market conditions. After 1996, as required by the Charities Act 1993, the Investment Fund disappears. It was analysed and divided into three, Endowment, Scholarship Investment Reserve and General Investment Reserve. Scholarship funds, although *designated*, i.e. set aside for a specific purpose, are disbursed at the trustees discretion and are *unrestricted*. The general fund alone, although shrunk to £2,497 in 1984, features every year.

Prior consultation is desired with any donor wishing to restrict the trustees' discretion over the manner, or beneficial region, in which funds, they wish to donate for the award of training grants, may be disbursed.

Appendix G

Societies Represented by Students

As reported on the charity's 90th Anniversary Programme, the names printed in italics would not be included but for the fact they represent a name no longer in current use (marked *).

Acre Gospel Mission
Action Partners was SUM
Afghan Border Crusade*
Africa Evangelical Fellowship was SAGM
Africa Inland Mission
Algiers Mission Board
All Nations Christian College
Arab World Ministries
Assemblies of God
Baptist Missionary Society
Belgium Evangelical Mission (BGM)
Belgium Gospel Mission*
Bible Baptist Missionary Movement
Bible Churchmans Missionary Soc*
Board of World Mission & Unity was CSMS
Bolivian Inland Mission
British Syria Mission*
Central Asian Mission*
China Inland Mission now OMF
Christian Missions in Many Lands
Christian Outreach
Christian Medical Fellowship
Church Missionary Society
Church Mission to the Jews*
Church of England Zennana Medical Soc*
Church of Scotland Missionary Soc
Church of Sweden Missionary Soc
Church's Ministry Among Jews was CMJ
Colonial Mission*
Congo Evangelistic Mission*
Crosslinks was BCMS
Dohnavur Fellowship
Dravidian Mission*
Echoes of Service
Edinburgh Medical Missionary Society
Egypt General Mission
Evangelical Mission of South America
Finnish Free Missionary Society

German Missionary Fellowship
Grace Baptist Mission was SBM
HCJB-UK was WRMF
Heart of Africa Mission*
Holiness Mission*
Iglesia Anglicana en el Norte Argentino
Independent New Church
India North West Mission
International Christian Fellowship
Interserve was ZBMM
Irish Baptist Foreign Mission*
Japan Evangelistic Band
Jungle Tribes Mission*
Latin Link was RBMU
Lifeline Network International
London Missionary Society
Mambilima Mission Hospital
Medair
Mercy Ships
Methodist Church Overseas Division was MMS
Methodist Missionary Society*
Middle East Christian Outreach was BSM
Missão Evangélica Aos Índios do Brasil
Mission Aviation Fellowship
Moravian Mission*
New Testament Missionary Union
New Tribes Mission
North Africa Mission*
Northwest Frontier Fellowship was ABC
Norwegian Lutheran Mission
Norwegian Pentecostal Mission
NW Frontier Fellowship (ABC)
NW Kiangsi Mission*
Nyassa Industrial Mission*
Operation Mobilisation
Overseas Missionary Fellowship was CIM
Peru Inland Mission*
Poona & India Mission*

Qua Iboe Fellowship
Red Sea Mission*
Regions Beyond Missionary Union*
Salvation Army
Servants to Asia's Urban Poor
Seventh Day Adventists
SIM International was ICF & PIM
South Africa General Mission
South American Missionary Society
South Seas Evangelical Mission*
Southern Morocco Mission*
Spanish Gospel Mission
Strict Baptist Mission*
Sudan United Mission
Swedish Baptist Mission
Swiss Evangelical Brotherhood
Swiss India Mission

TEAM was RSM
Tear Fund
UFM Worldwide was UFM
Unevangelised Fields Mission*
United Society for the Propagation of The Gospel
Universities Mission to Central Africa*
WEC International was HAM & WEC
Westcott Mission*
World Radio Missionary Fellowship*
World Outreach Media
Worldwide Evangelisation Crusade*
Wycliffe Bible Translators
Youth With A Mission
Zambesi Industrial Mission
Zenana Bible & Medical Mission*

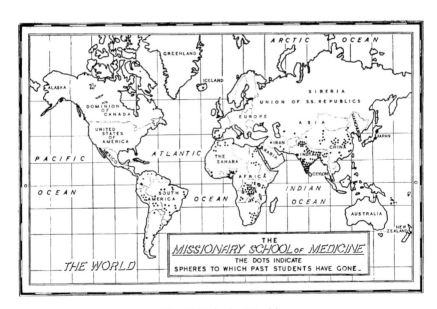

The Field is the World

And Jesus called his twelve disciples together ... and he sent them to preach the Kingdom of God and to heal the sick.
Luke 9: 1 & 2.

And they departed and went ... preaching the gospel and healing everywhere.
Luke 9: 6.

From the 50th annual report with the footnote,

The dots indicate the spheres to which approximately 1,300 past students
have gone forth to preach and heal.

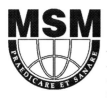

Statement of Faith

As an affiliate of Global Connections (EMA), Medical Service Ministries, its Staff, graduates and Grantees confess the historic Christian faith of the gospel of our Lord and Saviour, Jesus Christ.

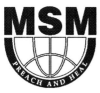

The sovereignty and grace of the triune God, Father, Son and Holy Spirit, in creation, providence, revelation, redemption and final judgment.

The divine inspiration and infallibility of the Old and New Testaments as originally given and their consequent entire trustworthiness and supreme authority in all matters of faith and conduct.

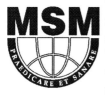

The universal sinfulness and guilt of fallen humankind deserving God's wrath and condemnation.

The substitutionary sacrifice of Jesus Christ, the incarnate Son of God, as the sole and all-sufficient ground of redemption from the guilt and power of sin and from its eternal consequences.

The justification of the sinner solely by the grace of God through faith in Christ

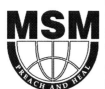

who was crucified and bodily raised from the dead.

The illuminating, regenerating, indwelling and sanctifying work of God the Holy Spirit. The priesthood of all believers, who form the universal Church, the Body of which Christ is the Head, and which is committed by his command to the proclamation of the gospel throughout the world.

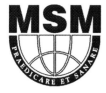

The expectation of the personal, visible return of the Lord Jesus Christ in power and glory.

Index

Index